NUTRIENT RICH FOODS

IFEANYICHUKWU EZEKWEM

CONTENTS

Book Overview

The book "Nutrient Rich Foods" provides a comprehensive guide to understanding and incorporating nutrient-rich foods into your diet. In the introduction, you will learn about the importance of nutrient-rich foods and how they can positively impact your overall health and well-being. The book explores the benefits of consuming nutrient-rich foods, such as improved energy levels, enhanced immune function, and better digestion. It also delves into the key nutrients that are essential for optimal health and explains how to incorporate them into your daily meals.

One of the key focuses of the book is on antioxidant-rich foods and superfoods. You will discover the power of antioxidants in fighting free radicals and reducing the risk of chronic diseases. The book provides a list of antioxidant-rich foods and superfoods, along with their specific health benefits. From berries and leafy greens to turmeric and chia seeds, you will learn about a wide range of nutrient-dense foods that can boost your health and vitality.

In addition to fruits and vegetables, the book explores the importance of incorporating whole grains into your diet. You will learn about the different types of whole grains and their nutritional benefits. The book also emphasizes the significance of lean protein sources, such as poultry, fish, and legumes, in providing essential amino acids for muscle repair and growth. Furthermore, it discusses the role of healthy fats, dairy, and dairy alternatives in supporting brain function and maintaining healthy bones.

The book "Nutrient Rich Foods" also provides practical tips for nutrient-rich snacking and meal planning. It explains the concept of nutrient density versus caloric density and how to make informed choices when it comes to food selection. Additionally, the book addresses the needs of individuals following special diets, such as vegetarian, vegan, or gluten-free, and offers suggestions for incorporating nutrient-rich foods into these dietary patterns. With a comprehensive list of references, the book ensures that you have access to reliable sources for further exploration of the topic.

free, and offers suggestions for incorporating nutrient-rich foods into these dietary patterns. With a comprehensive list of references, the book ensures that you have access to reliable sources for further exploration of the topic.

INTRODUCTION TO NUTRIENT RICH FOODS

Understanding Nutrient Rich Foods

Nutrient rich foods are those that provide a high concentration of essential nutrients, such as vitamins, minerals, fiber, and antioxidants, while being relatively low in calories. These foods are often referred to as "superfoods" because of their exceptional nutritional value and health benefits. Understanding the concept of nutrient rich foods is crucial for making informed dietary choices and optimizing your overall health and well-being.

When we talk about nutrient rich foods, we are referring to a wide variety of fruits, vegetables, whole grains, lean proteins, healthy fats, and dairy or dairy alternatives that are packed with essential nutrients. These foods are not only rich in vitamins and minerals but also contain other beneficial compounds like antioxidants and phytochemicals, which have been shown to have numerous health-promoting effects.

To better understand the concept of nutrient rich foods, let's take a closer look at some examples:

.

Fruits and Vegetables: Fruits and vegetables are the cornerstone of a nutrient rich diet. They are packed with vitamins, minerals, fiber, and antioxidants. For example, berries like blueberries and strawberries are rich in antioxidants, while leafy greens like spinach and kale are excellent sources of vitamins A, C, and K.

.

.

Whole Grains: Whole grains, such as quinoa, brown rice, and oats, are nutrient rich alternatives to refined grains. They are high in fiber, B vitamins, and minerals like magnesium and selenium. These grains provide sustained energy and help regulate blood sugar levels.

.

.

Lean Proteins: Lean proteins, such as chicken, turkey, fish, tofu, and legumes, are excellent sources of essential amino acids, which are the building blocks of proteins. They also provide important nutrients like iron, zinc, and B vitamins. Including lean proteins in your diet helps support muscle growth, repair, and overall health.

.

.

Healthy Fats: Healthy fats, such as avocados, nuts, seeds, and olive oil, are essential for optimal health. They provide essential fatty acids, like omega-3 and omega-6, which are important for brain function, heart health, and reducing inflammation. Including these fats in moderation can help improve nutrient absorption and promote satiety.

.

.

Dairy and Dairy Alternatives: Dairy products like milk, yogurt, and cheese are excellent sources of calcium, vitamin D, and protein. However, if you are lactose intolerant or follow a vegan diet, there are plenty of dairy alternatives available, such as almond milk, soy milk, and coconut yogurt, that can provide similar nutrients.

.

By incorporating these nutrient rich foods into your diet, you can ensure that you are getting a wide range of essential nutrients to support your overall health and well-being. It's important to note that nutrient rich foods are not limited to these examples, and there are many other options available depending on your dietary preferences and needs.

Understanding the concept of nutrient density is also crucial when discussing nutrient rich foods. Nutrient density refers to the amount of nutrients per calorie in a particular food. Foods that are nutrient dense provide a high amount of essential nutrients relative to their calorie content. For example, a handful of nuts may be high in calories, but they also provide a significant amount of vitamins, minerals, and healthy fats, making them a nutrient dense choice.

In contrast, foods that are calorie dense but low in nutrients, such as sugary snacks and processed foods, are considered to have low nutrient density. These foods often provide empty calories, meaning they contribute to weight gain without offering much in terms of essential nutrients.

Understanding the concept of nutrient density can help you make informed food choices and prioritize nutrient rich foods in your diet. By focusing on nutrient dense options, you can ensure that you are getting the most nutritional bang for your buck and supporting your overall health and well-being.

In the next section, we will explore the importance of a nutrient rich diet and how it can positively impact your health.

The Importance of a Nutrient Rich Diet

A nutrient-rich diet is essential for maintaining optimal health and well-being. It provides the body with the necessary vitamins, minerals, antioxidants, and other essential nutrients that are required for various bodily functions. Consuming a diet rich in nutrients can have numerous benefits, including improved energy levels, enhanced immune function, better digestion, and a reduced risk of chronic diseases.

One of the primary reasons why a nutrient-rich diet is important is because it provides the body with the fuel it needs to function properly. Nutrients are the building blocks of our bodies, and they play a crucial role in maintaining the health of our cells, tissues, and organs. For example, vitamins and minerals are essential for the proper functioning of our immune system, which helps protect us from infections and diseases.

A nutrient-rich diet also helps to support optimal growth and development, especially in children and adolescents. During these stages of life, the body requires a higher intake of nutrients to support the growth of bones, muscles, and organs. Adequate intake of nutrients such as calcium, vitamin D, and protein is crucial for the development of strong bones and muscles.

Furthermore, a nutrient-rich diet can help to prevent and manage chronic diseases. Many chronic diseases, such as heart disease, diabetes, and certain types of cancer, are often linked to poor dietary choices and a lack of essential nutrients. By consuming a diet rich in fruits, vegetables, whole grains, lean proteins, and healthy fats, individuals can reduce their risk of developing these diseases and improve their overall health.

For example, a diet high in fruits and vegetables has been associated with a lower risk of heart disease and stroke. These foods are rich in antioxidants, which help to protect the body against oxidative stress and inflammation, both of which are risk factors for cardiovascular diseases. Additionally, the fiber found in fruits and vegetables can help to lower cholesterol levels and regulate blood sugar levels, reducing the risk of diabetes.

Incorporating nutrient-rich foods into your diet can also help to maintain a healthy weight. Nutrient-dense foods are typically lower in calories but higher in essential nutrients, which means that you can consume a larger volume of food while still meeting your nutritional needs. This can help to prevent overeating and promote satiety, making it easier to maintain a healthy weight.

For example, choosing whole grains over refined grains can help to increase satiety and reduce the risk of overeating. Whole grains are rich in fiber, which slows down digestion and keeps you feeling fuller for longer. On the other hand, refined grains, such as white bread and white rice, are stripped of their fiber content and can cause blood sugar spikes, leading to cravings and overeating.

In addition to the physical benefits, a nutrient-rich diet can also have a positive impact on mental health. Research has shown that certain nutrients, such as omega-3 fatty acids found in fatty fish, can help to improve mood and reduce the risk of depression. Other nutrients, such as B vitamins and magnesium, are also important for brain health and cognitive function.

Incorporating a variety of nutrient-rich foods into your diet is key to reaping the benefits. Aim to include a wide range of fruits, vegetables, whole grains, lean proteins, and healthy fats in your meals and snacks. For example, instead of reaching for a bag of chips as a snack, opt for a handful of nuts or a piece of fruit. Swap out processed foods for whole foods whenever possible, and experiment with different recipes and cooking methods to make your meals more nutritious and enjoyable.

In conclusion, a nutrient-rich diet is of utmost importance for maintaining optimal health and well-being. It provides the body with the necessary nutrients to support various bodily functions, promote growth and development, prevent chronic diseases, maintain a healthy weight, and support mental health. By incorporating a variety of nutrient-rich foods into your diet, you can enhance your overall health and improve your quality of life.

How Nutrient Rich Foods

Benefit Your Health

Nutrient rich foods are an essential component of a healthy diet. They provide the body with the necessary vitamins, minerals, antioxidants, and other important nutrients needed for optimal health and well-being. Incorporating nutrient rich foods into your diet can have numerous benefits for your overall health. In this section, we will explore how nutrient rich foods benefit your health and provide you with some relatable examples.

1. Improved Energy Levels

One of the primary benefits of consuming nutrient rich foods is improved energy levels. Nutrient rich foods are packed with vitamins, minerals, and complex carbohydrates that provide a steady release of energy throughout the day. For example, foods such as whole grains, fruits, and vegetables are rich in fiber and slow-digesting carbohydrates, which help to stabilize blood sugar levels and provide sustained energy. By incorporating these foods into your diet, you can avoid energy crashes and maintain a consistent level of energy throughout the day.

2. Enhanced Immune Function

A strong immune system is crucial for fighting off infections and diseases. Nutrient rich foods play a vital role in supporting and enhancing immune function. For instance, foods rich in vitamin C, such as citrus fruits, berries, and leafy greens, can boost the production of white blood cells, which are essential for fighting off pathogens. Additionally, foods high in zinc, such as lean meats, seafood, and legumes, can help strengthen the immune system and promote the production of antibodies. By incorporating these nutrient rich foods into your diet, you can give your immune system the support it needs to function optimally.

3. Improved Digestive Health

A healthy digestive system is essential for nutrient absorption and overall well-being. Nutrient rich foods, particularly those high in fiber, can promote good digestive health. Fiber helps to regulate bowel movements, prevent constipation, and maintain a healthy gut microbiome. Examples of fiber-rich foods include whole grains, legumes, fruits, and vegetables. By including these foods in your diet, you can support a healthy digestive system and improve nutrient absorption.

4. Reduced Risk of Chronic Diseases

A diet rich in nutrients has been associated with a reduced risk of chronic diseases such as heart disease, diabetes, and certain types of cancer. Nutrient rich foods are typically low in unhealthy fats, added sugars, and sodium, which are known to contribute to the development of these diseases. Instead, they are packed with antioxidants, phytochemicals, and other bioactive compounds that have been shown to have protective effects against chronic diseases. For example, foods such as berries, leafy greens, and nuts are rich in antioxidants that can help reduce inflammation and oxidative stress, both of which are linked to chronic diseases. By incorporating these nutrient rich foods into your diet, you can lower your risk of developing these conditions and promote long-term health.

5. Weight Management

Maintaining a healthy weight is important for overall health and well-being. Nutrient rich foods can play a significant role in weight management. These foods are typically low in calories but high in nutrients, which means you can consume larger portions without consuming excessive calories. For example, a large salad made with leafy greens, colorful vegetables, and lean protein can be filling and satisfying while providing a wide range of essential nutrients. By incorporating nutrient rich foods into your meals, you can feel satisfied and nourished while managing your weight effectively.

6. Improved Cognitive Function

Nutrient rich foods are not only beneficial for the body but also for the brain. Certain nutrients, such as omega-3 fatty acids, vitamins B6 and B12, and antioxidants, have been shown to support brain health and cognitive function. For instance, fatty fish like salmon and trout are rich in omega-3 fatty acids, which are essential for brain development and function. Leafy greens, berries, and nuts are also known to have cognitive benefits due to their high antioxidant content. By including these nutrient rich foods in your diet, you can support brain health and potentially reduce the risk of cognitive decline.

7. Improved Mood and Mental Well-being

The food we eat can have a significant impact on our mood and mental well-being. Nutrient rich foods can help support a positive mood and mental health. For example, foods rich in omega-3 fatty acids, such as fatty fish, walnuts, and flaxseeds, have been shown to have mood-enhancing effects. Additionally, foods high in B vitamins, such as whole grains, legumes, and leafy greens, can support the production of neurotransmitters that regulate mood, such as serotonin and dopamine. By incorporating these nutrient rich foods into your diet, you can support a healthy mood and overall mental well-being.

Incorporating nutrient rich foods into your diet can have a profound impact on your health and well-being. From improved energy levels to reduced risk of chronic diseases, the benefits are numerous. By making conscious choices to include nutrient rich foods in your meals and snacks, you can nourish your body and support optimal health.

Incorporating Nutrient Rich Foods into Your Diet

Incorporating nutrient-rich foods into your diet is essential for maintaining optimal health and well-being. These foods are packed with vitamins, minerals, antioxidants, and other essential nutrients that support various bodily functions and help prevent chronic diseases. By making conscious choices and incorporating these foods into your daily meals, you can ensure that your body receives the nourishment it needs to thrive.

Here are some practical tips and strategies to help you incorporate nutrient-rich foods into your diet:

- **Plan your meals:** Meal planning is a great way to ensure that you have a variety of nutrient-rich foods in your diet. Take some time each week to plan your meals and create a shopping list. Include a mix of fruits, vegetables, whole grains, lean proteins, and healthy fats in your plan. This will not only help you stay organized but also ensure that you have the necessary ingredients on hand to prepare nutritious meals.

- **Start with small changes:** Incorporating nutrient-rich foods into your diet doesn't have to be overwhelming. Start by making small changes to your meals. For example, swap out refined grains for whole grains, replace sugary snacks with fresh fruits, or choose lean proteins like chicken or fish instead of processed meats. These small changes can add up over time and make a significant difference in your overall nutrient intake.

- **Experiment with new recipes:** Trying out new recipes can be a fun and exciting way to incorporate nutrient-rich foods into your diet. Look for recipes that feature a variety of fruits, vegetables, whole grains, and lean proteins. Experiment with different flavors, spices, and cooking techniques to keep your meals interesting and enjoyable. There are countless online resources and cookbooks available that provide nutritious and delicious recipes to suit every taste.

- **Make smart substitutions:** Another effective way to incorporate nutrient-rich foods into your diet is by making smart substitutions. For example, instead of using butter or margarine, try spreading avocado or nut butter on your toast. Swap out sugary drinks for herbal teas or infused water. Replace high-fat salad dressings with homemade vinaigrettes made with olive oil and vinegar. These simple substitutions can significantly increase the nutrient content of your meals without sacrificing taste.

.

.

Include a variety of colors: One way to ensure that you're getting a wide range of nutrients is by including a variety of colors in your meals. Different colored fruits and vegetables contain different vitamins, minerals, and antioxidants. Aim to include a rainbow of colors on your plate, such as red tomatoes, orange carrots, green spinach, and purple berries. This not only makes your meals visually appealing but also ensures that you're getting a diverse range of nutrients.

.

.

Snack smartly: Snacking can be an opportunity to incorporate nutrient-rich foods into your diet. Instead of reaching for processed snacks like chips or cookies, opt for healthier alternatives such as fresh fruits, raw nuts, or yogurt. These snacks provide essential nutrients and can help keep you satisfied between meals. Prepare snack packs in advance to have them readily available when hunger strikes.

.

.

Be mindful of portion sizes: While incorporating nutrient-rich foods into your diet is important, it's also essential to be mindful of portion sizes. Even healthy foods can contribute to weight gain if consumed in excess. Pay attention to your body's hunger and fullness cues and practice portion control. Balancing your nutrient intake with your caloric needs is key to maintaining a healthy weight and overall well-being.

.

.

Stay hydrated: Hydration is often overlooked but plays a crucial role in overall health. Make sure to drink an adequate amount of water throughout the day. You can also incorporate hydrating foods into your diet, such as watermelon, cucumbers, and leafy greens. Staying hydrated helps your body absorb and utilize nutrients effectively.

.

Remember, incorporating nutrient-rich foods into your diet is a journey, and it's important to be patient with yourself. Gradually make changes and find what works best for you. By prioritizing nutrient-rich foods and making conscious choices, you can nourish your body and enjoy the benefits of a healthy and vibrant life.

KEY NUTRIENTS

Essential Vitamins for Optimal Health

Vitamins are essential nutrients that our bodies need in small amounts to function properly. They play a crucial role in maintaining overall health and well-being. While a balanced diet should provide us with an adequate amount of vitamins, it is important to understand the specific vitamins our bodies need and the benefits they provide.

Vitamin A

Vitamin A is a fat-soluble vitamin that is important for maintaining healthy vision, promoting growth and development, and supporting the immune system. It is found in foods such as carrots, sweet potatoes, spinach, and liver. Vitamin A is also important for the health of our skin and mucous membranes, which act as a barrier against bacteria and viruses.

Vitamin B Complex

The B vitamins are a group of water-soluble vitamins that play a vital role in energy production, brain function, and the formation of red blood cells. They include thiamine (B1), riboflavin (B2), niacin (B3), pantothenic acid (B5), pyridoxine (B6), biotin (B7), folate (B9), and cobalamin (B12). Each B vitamin has its own specific functions, but they often work together to support overall health. Good sources of B vitamins include whole grains, legumes, leafy greens, eggs, and lean meats.

Vitamin C

Vitamin C, also known as ascorbic acid, is a water-soluble vitamin that acts as an antioxidant in the body. It is important for the growth, development, and repair of all body tissues. Vitamin C also helps in the production of collagen, a protein that is essential for the health of our skin, bones, and blood vessels. Citrus fruits, strawberries, bell peppers, and broccoli are excellent sources of vitamin C.

Vitamin D

Vitamin D is a unique vitamin because our bodies can produce it when our skin is exposed to sunlight. It is also found in certain foods such as fatty fish, fortified dairy products, and egg yolks. Vitamin D plays a crucial role in calcium absorption, which is essential for maintaining strong bones and teeth. It also supports immune function and helps regulate cell growth and division.

Vitamin E

Vitamin E is a fat-soluble vitamin that acts as an antioxidant, protecting our cells from damage caused by free radicals. It also plays a role in immune function and the formation of red blood cells. Good sources of vitamin E include nuts, seeds, vegetable oils, and leafy greens.

Vitamin K

Vitamin K is a fat-soluble vitamin that is important for blood clotting and bone health. It helps in the synthesis of proteins that are involved in blood clotting, preventing excessive bleeding. Vitamin K is also necessary for the proper mineralization of bones, which helps maintain their strength.

Leafy greens, broccoli, and Brussels sprouts are excellent sources of vitamin K.

Importance of a Balanced Vitamin Intake

Each vitamin plays a unique role in our bodies, and a deficiency in any one of them can lead to specific health problems. For example, a deficiency in vitamin A can cause night blindness and an increased susceptibility to infections. Vitamin C deficiency can lead to scurvy, a disease characterized by fatigue, bleeding gums, and poor wound healing. Vitamin D deficiency can result in weakened bones and an increased risk of fractures.

On the other hand, consuming excessive amounts of certain vitamins can also have negative effects on our health. For instance, an excess of vitamin A can lead to toxicity symptoms such as nausea, dizziness, and even hair loss. It is important to maintain a balanced intake of vitamins through a varied and nutrient-rich diet.

Incorporating a wide range of fruits, vegetables, whole grains, lean proteins, and healthy fats into our meals can help ensure that we are getting an adequate amount of vitamins. It is also important to note that some vitamins are more easily absorbed when consumed with certain foods. For example, vitamin C enhances the absorption of iron from plant-based sources, so pairing foods rich in vitamin C with iron-rich foods can optimize iron absorption.

In conclusion, essential vitamins are vital for optimal health and well-being. They support various bodily functions and help prevent deficiencies and related health problems. By incorporating a diverse range of nutrient-rich foods into our diets, we can ensure that we are getting an adequate amount of vitamins to support our overall health.

Minerals and Their Role in a Nutrient Rich Diet

Minerals are essential nutrients that play a crucial role in maintaining overall health and well-being. They are inorganic substances that our bodies need in small amounts to function properly. While minerals are not a source of energy like carbohydrates, proteins, and fats, they are involved in various physiological processes and are vital for the proper functioning of our body systems.

Minerals can be divided into two categories: macrominerals and trace minerals. Macrominerals are required in larger amounts, while trace minerals are needed in smaller quantities. Both types of minerals are equally important for maintaining optimal health.

Macrominerals

Macrominerals are minerals that our bodies need in larger amounts. They include calcium, phosphorus, magnesium, sodium, potassium, and chloride. Let's explore the role of each macromineral in a nutrient-rich diet:

-

Calcium: Calcium is well-known for its role in maintaining strong bones and teeth. It also plays a crucial role in muscle function, nerve transmission, and blood clotting. Good sources of calcium include dairy products, leafy green vegetables, tofu, and fortified plant-based milk alternatives.

-

Phosphorus: Phosphorus works closely with calcium to build and maintain healthy bones and teeth. It is also involved in energy production, DNA synthesis, and cell repair. Good sources of phosphorus include dairy products, meat, fish, poultry, nuts, and legumes.

-

-

Magnesium: Magnesium is involved in over 300 biochemical reactions in the body. It plays a vital role in muscle and nerve function, blood pressure regulation, and energy production. Good sources of magnesium include leafy green vegetables, whole grains, nuts, seeds, and legumes.

.

.

Sodium: Sodium is necessary for maintaining fluid balance, nerve function, and muscle contraction. However, excessive sodium intake can contribute to high blood pressure. It is important to consume sodium in moderation and choose sources that are low in added salt. Natural sources of sodium include vegetables, fruits, dairy products, and small amounts found in whole grains and legumes.

.

.

Potassium: Potassium works in conjunction with sodium to maintain fluid balance and regulate blood pressure. It is also involved in muscle contractions and nerve function. Good sources of potassium include bananas, oranges, leafy green vegetables, potatoes, and legumes.

.

.

Chloride: Chloride is an essential mineral that helps maintain fluid balance, aids in digestion, and is involved in the production of stomach acid. It is found in table salt and many processed foods. Natural sources of chloride include seaweed, tomatoes, lettuce, and olives.

.

Trace Minerals

Trace minerals are required in smaller amounts but are equally important for overall health. They include iron, zinc, copper, manganese, iodine, selenium, and molybdenum. Let's explore the role of each trace mineral in a nutrient-rich diet:

.

Iron: Iron is essential for the production of hemoglobin, a protein in red blood cells that carries oxygen throughout the body. It is also involved in energy production and immune function. Good sources of iron include lean meats, poultry, fish, legumes, fortified cereals, and leafy green vegetables.

.

.

Zinc: Zinc is involved in numerous enzymatic reactions in the body and plays a crucial role in immune function, wound healing, and DNA synthesis. Good sources of zinc include oysters, beef, poultry, dairy products, nuts, and legumes.

.

.

Copper: Copper is necessary for the formation of red blood cells, collagen production, and iron absorption. It also acts as an antioxidant, protecting cells from damage. Good sources of copper include organ meats, shellfish, nuts, seeds, and whole grains.

.

.

Manganese: Manganese is involved in bone formation, metabolism, and antioxidant defense. It also plays a role in the production of collagen and cartilage. Good sources of manganese include whole grains, nuts, seeds, legumes, and leafy green vegetables.

.

.

Iodine: Iodine is essential for the production of thyroid hormones, which regulate metabolism and growth. Good sources of iodine include iodized salt, seafood, seaweed, and dairy products.

.

.

Selenium: Selenium is a powerful antioxidant that helps protect cells from damage. It also plays a role in thyroid function and immune system health. Good sources of selenium include Brazil nuts, seafood, poultry, meat, and whole grains.

.

.

Molybdenum: Molybdenum is involved in various enzymatic

reactions in the body and plays a role in the metabolism of certain amino acids. Good sources of molybdenum include legumes, whole grains, leafy green vegetables, and organ meats.

.

Incorporating a variety of nutrient-rich foods into your diet ensures an adequate intake of essential minerals. By including foods rich in macrominerals and trace minerals, you can support optimal health and well-being. Remember to consult with a healthcare professional or registered dietitian for personalized advice based on your specific dietary needs.

The Power of Fiber in Nutrient Rich Foods

Fiber is an essential component of a nutrient-rich diet that often goes unnoticed. While it may not receive as much attention as other nutrients, such as vitamins and minerals, fiber plays a crucial role in maintaining optimal health and well-being. In this section, we will explore the power of fiber in nutrient-rich foods and how it contributes to overall health.

Understanding Fiber

Fiber is a type of carbohydrate that cannot be digested by the human body. It passes through the digestive system relatively intact, providing a range of health benefits along the way. There are two main types of fiber: soluble and insoluble.

Soluble fiber dissolves in water and forms a gel-like substance in the digestive tract. It can help lower cholesterol levels, regulate blood sugar levels, and promote a feeling of fullness, which can aid in weight management. Good sources of soluble fiber include oats, barley, legumes, fruits, and vegetables.

Insoluble fiber, on the other hand, does not dissolve in water and adds bulk to the stool. It helps prevent constipation, promotes regular bowel movements, and supports a healthy digestive system. Whole grains, nuts, seeds, and the skin of fruits and vegetables are excellent sources of insoluble fiber.

The Health Benefits of Fiber

Including fiber-rich foods in your diet can have numerous

health benefits. Here are some of the key advantages of consuming a diet high in fiber:

.

Improved Digestive Health: Fiber adds bulk to the stool, making it easier to pass through the digestive system. This can help prevent constipation and promote regular bowel movements, reducing the risk of digestive disorders such as hemorrhoids, diverticulitis, and irritable bowel syndrome.

.

.

Weight Management: High-fiber foods tend to be more filling, which can help control appetite and prevent overeating. Additionally, fiber-rich foods often require more chewing, which slows down the eating process and allows the body to register feelings of fullness more effectively.

.

.

Heart Health: Soluble fiber has been shown to help lower LDL (bad) cholesterol levels, reducing the risk of heart disease. It does this by binding to cholesterol in the digestive system and preventing its absorption into the bloodstream. Good sources of soluble fiber, such as oats and legumes, can be particularly beneficial for heart health.

.

.

Blood Sugar Control: Soluble fiber can help regulate blood sugar levels by slowing down the absorption of glucose into the bloodstream. This can be especially beneficial for individuals with diabetes or those at risk of developing the condition.

.

.

Reduced Risk of Chronic Diseases: A diet high in fiber has been associated with a lower risk of developing various chronic diseases, including type 2 diabetes, certain types of cancer (such as colorectal cancer), and cardiovascular disease.

.

Incorporating Fiber into Your Diet

Now that we understand the importance of fiber in a nutrient-rich diet, let's explore some practical ways to incorporate more fiber-rich foods into your meals:

- **Choose Whole Grains**: Opt for whole grain bread, pasta, and rice instead of their refined counterparts. Whole grains retain the bran and germ, which are rich in fiber, vitamins, and minerals.

- **Include Fruits and Vegetables**: Aim to include a variety of fruits and vegetables in your daily meals. Leave the skin on whenever possible, as it contains a significant amount of fiber.

- **Snack on Nuts and Seeds**: Nuts and seeds, such as almonds, chia seeds, and flaxseeds, are not only rich in healthy fats but also provide a good amount of fiber. Enjoy them as a snack or sprinkle them on top of salads, yogurt, or oatmeal.

- **Add Legumes to Your Diet**: Legumes, including beans, lentils, and chickpeas, are excellent sources of both soluble and insoluble fiber. Incorporate them into soups, stews, salads, or even as a meat substitute in dishes like chili or tacos.

- **Choose High-Fiber Snacks**: Opt for snacks that are naturally high in fiber, such as fresh fruits, raw vegetables, whole grain crackers, or air-popped popcorn.

- **Read Food Labels**: When purchasing packaged foods, check the nutrition labels for the fiber content. Choose products that have a higher fiber content per serving.

Remember to increase your fiber intake gradually and drink plenty of water throughout the day. This will help prevent any digestive discomfort that may arise from a sudden increase in fiber consumption.

In conclusion, fiber is a powerful nutrient that plays a vital role in maintaining optimal health. By incorporating fiber-rich foods into your diet, you can support digestive health, manage weight, promote heart health, regulate blood sugar levels, and reduce the risk of chronic diseases. So, make sure to include a variety of fiber-rich foods in your meals and enjoy the numerous health benefits they provide.

Protein

Protein is an essential nutrient that plays a crucial role in our overall health and well-being. It is often referred to as the building block of life, as it is responsible for the growth, repair, and maintenance of tissues in our body. Protein is made up of amino acids, which are the building blocks of protein molecules. There are 20 different amino acids, and our body needs all of them to function properly.

Protein is found in a variety of foods, both animal and plant-based. Animal sources of protein include meat, poultry, fish, eggs, and dairy products. These sources are considered complete proteins because they contain all the essential amino acids that our body needs. Plant-based sources of protein include legumes, nuts, seeds, and grains. While these sources may not contain all the essential amino acids, they can still provide an adequate amount of protein when combined with other plant-based foods.

Including protein-rich foods in our diet is important for several reasons. Firstly, protein is essential for muscle growth and repair. When we engage in physical activity or exercise, our muscles undergo stress and damage. Protein helps in repairing and rebuilding these muscles, allowing them to grow stronger and more resilient. This is particularly important for athletes and individuals who engage in regular exercise.

Protein also plays a crucial role in maintaining a healthy immune system. Our immune system relies on proteins to produce antibodies, which are proteins that help fight off infections and diseases. Without an adequate amount of protein, our immune system may become compromised, making us more susceptible to illnesses.

In addition to its role in muscle growth and immune function, protein is also important for maintaining healthy skin, hair, and nails. The proteins collagen and keratin are responsible for the strength and elasticity of our skin, hair, and nails. Including protein-rich foods in our diet can help promote healthy skin, reduce the risk of hair loss, and strengthen our nails.

Protein is also known for its satiating effect, meaning it helps keep us feeling full and satisfied after a meal. This can be particularly beneficial for individuals who are trying to lose weight or maintain a healthy weight. Including protein-rich foods in our meals can help curb cravings and prevent overeating, ultimately supporting our weight management goals.

When it comes to protein intake, the recommended daily amount varies depending on factors such as age, sex, and activity level. The general guideline is to consume about 0.8 grams of protein per kilogram of body weight. However, athletes and individuals who engage in intense physical activity may require higher amounts of protein to support muscle repair and growth.

It's important to note that while protein is an essential nutrient, it should be consumed in moderation. Excessive protein intake can put strain on the kidneys and may lead to health issues in the long term. It's always best to consult with a healthcare professional or registered dietitian to determine the appropriate amount of protein for your individual needs.

Incorporating protein-rich foods into our diet can be done in a variety of ways. For those who consume animal products, lean meats such as chicken, turkey, and fish are excellent sources of protein. Eggs and dairy products like Greek yogurt and cottage cheese are also rich in protein. Plant-based sources of protein include legumes such as lentils, chickpeas, and black beans, as well as nuts, seeds, and whole grains like quinoa and brown rice. Here are a few examples of protein-rich meals and snacks:

- Grilled chicken breast with steamed vegetables and quinoa
- Greek yogurt topped with berries and a sprinkle of nuts
- Lentil soup with a side of whole grain bread
- Tofu stir-fry with mixed vegetables and brown rice
- Hard-boiled eggs with avocado on whole grain toast

By incorporating protein-rich foods into our meals and snacks, we can ensure that we are meeting our body's protein needs and reaping the many benefits that protein has to offer. Whether we choose animal or plant-based sources of protein, it's important to prioritize this nutrient in our diet for optimal health and well-being.

ANTIOXIDANT RICH FOODS

Understanding Antioxidants and Their Benefits

Antioxidants have gained significant attention in recent years for their potential health benefits. But what exactly are antioxidants, and why are they so important for our well-being? In this section, we will delve into the world of antioxidants, exploring their role in the body and the numerous benefits they offer.

What are Antioxidants?

Antioxidants are compounds that help protect our cells from damage caused by harmful molecules called free radicals. Free radicals are highly reactive molecules that can be generated through various processes in the body, such as metabolism or exposure to environmental factors like pollution or UV radiation. When free radicals accumulate in the body, they can cause oxidative stress, leading to cellular damage and potentially contributing to the development of chronic diseases. Antioxidants work by neutralizing free radicals, preventing them from causing harm to our cells. They do this by donating an electron to the free radicals, effectively stabilizing them and reducing their damaging effects. Antioxidants can be found in a wide range of foods, particularly in fruits, vegetables, nuts, seeds, and certain beverages like green tea.

The Benefits of Antioxidants

The consumption of antioxidant-rich foods has been associated with numerous health benefits. Let's explore some of the key advantages that antioxidants offer:

1. Protection against Chronic Diseases

Research suggests that a diet rich in antioxidants may help reduce the risk of chronic diseases, including heart disease, certain types of cancer, and neurodegenerative disorders like Alzheimer's and Parkinson's disease. By neutralizing free radicals, antioxidants help prevent cellular damage and inflammation, which are underlying factors in the development of these conditions.

2. Anti-Aging Effects

Oxidative stress and the accumulation of free radicals can contribute to the aging process. Antioxidants, by combating oxidative stress, may help slow down the aging process and promote healthier, more youthful-looking skin. They can also protect against age-related vision problems, such as macular degeneration.

3. Immune System Support

Antioxidants play a crucial role in supporting a healthy immune system. By neutralizing free radicals, they help reduce inflammation and enhance immune cell function, allowing the body to better defend against infections and diseases.

4. Cardiovascular Health

Antioxidants, particularly flavonoids found in fruits and vegetables, have been linked to improved cardiovascular health.

They can help lower blood pressure, reduce LDL cholesterol levels, and improve blood vessel function, all of which contribute to a healthier heart and a reduced risk of heart disease.

5. Eye Health

Certain antioxidants, such as lutein and zeaxanthin, are especially beneficial for eye health. They accumulate in the retina and help protect against age-related macular degeneration and cataracts, two common eye conditions that can lead to vision loss.

6. Cognitive Function

Oxidative stress and inflammation in the brain have been implicated in cognitive decline and neurodegenerative diseases. Antioxidants, by reducing oxidative stress and inflammation, may help preserve cognitive function and protect against conditions like Alzheimer's and dementia.

Food Sources of Antioxidants

To reap the benefits of antioxidants, it is important to incorporate a variety of antioxidant-rich foods into your diet. Here are some examples of foods that are particularly high in antioxidants:

- Berries: Blueberries, strawberries, raspberries, and blackberries are all excellent sources of antioxidants, particularly anthocyanins.
- Dark Chocolate: High-quality dark chocolate contains flavonoids and polyphenols, which have potent antioxidant properties.
- Leafy Greens: Spinach, kale, and Swiss chard are packed with antioxidants like vitamins C and E, as well as lutein and zeaxanthin.
- Nuts and Seeds: Almonds, walnuts, chia seeds, and flaxseeds are all rich in antioxidants, healthy fats, and other beneficial nutrients.
- Green Tea: Green tea is loaded with catechins, a type of antioxidant that has been linked to numerous

health benefits.

- Citrus Fruits: Oranges, lemons, and grapefruits are excellent sources of vitamin C, a powerful antioxidant.
- Tomatoes: Tomatoes contain lycopene, a potent antioxidant that gives them their vibrant red color.
- Red Wine: In moderation, red wine provides antioxidants like resveratrol, which has been associated with heart health benefits.

Conclusion

Antioxidants play a vital role in protecting our cells from damage and promoting overall health and well-being. By incorporating antioxidant-rich foods into our diet, we can harness the power of these compounds and enjoy their numerous benefits. From reducing the risk of chronic diseases to supporting a healthy immune system and promoting youthful skin, antioxidants are truly a cornerstone of a nutrient-rich diet. So, make sure to fill your plate with a colorful array of fruits, vegetables, nuts, seeds, and other antioxidant-rich foods to nourish your body and optimize your health.

Top Antioxidant Rich Foods and Their Health Benefits

Antioxidants play a crucial role in maintaining our overall health and well-being. They are compounds that help protect our cells from damage caused by harmful molecules called free radicals. Free radicals are produced naturally in our bodies as a result of various metabolic processes, but they can also be generated by external factors such as pollution, smoking, and exposure to radiation.

Consuming a diet rich in antioxidants is essential for neutralizing free radicals and reducing the risk of chronic diseases such as heart disease, cancer, and neurodegenerative disorders. Luckily, there are numerous antioxidant-rich foods that we can incorporate into our daily meals to boost our antioxidant intake. Let's explore some of the top antioxidant-rich foods and their specific health benefits:

Berries

Berries, such as blueberries, strawberries, raspberries, and blackberries, are packed with antioxidants known as anthocyanins. These compounds give berries their vibrant colors and offer a wide range of health benefits. Anthocyanins have been shown to reduce inflammation, improve cognitive function, and protect against age-related decline in brain function. Additionally, berries are rich in vitamin C, which further enhances their antioxidant properties and supports immune health.

Dark Chocolate

Yes, you read that right! Dark chocolate, specifically those with a high cocoa content (70% or more), is an excellent source of antioxidants. The cocoa beans used to make dark chocolate are rich in flavonoids, a type of antioxidant that has been linked to numerous health benefits. Flavonoids in dark chocolate have been shown to improve heart health by reducing blood pressure, improving blood flow, and reducing the risk of blood clots. However, it's important to consume dark chocolate in moderation due to its high calorie and fat content.

Green Leafy Vegetables

Green leafy vegetables, such as spinach, kale, and Swiss chard, are not only rich in vitamins and minerals but also in antioxidants. These vegetables contain a variety of antioxidants, including vitamin C, vitamin E, and beta-carotene. These antioxidants help protect our cells from damage, reduce inflammation, and support overall immune function. Incorporating a variety of green leafy vegetables into your diet can provide a significant boost to your antioxidant intake.

Nuts and Seeds

Nuts and seeds, such as almonds, walnuts, flaxseeds, and chia seeds, are not only a great source of healthy fats and protein but also contain high levels of antioxidants. These antioxidant-rich foods are particularly rich in vitamin E, which acts as a potent antioxidant in our bodies. Vitamin E helps protect our cells from oxidative damage, supports immune function, and may even reduce the risk of chronic diseases such as heart disease and certain types of cancer.

Colorful Vegetables and Fruits

Vibrantly colored vegetables and fruits, such as tomatoes, carrots, bell peppers, and oranges, are packed with antioxidants. These colorful foods contain a variety of antioxidants, including vitamin C, beta-carotene, and lycopene. Lycopene, found in tomatoes and watermelon, has been associated with a reduced risk of certain types of cancer, particularly prostate cancer. Including a rainbow of fruits and vegetables in your diet ensures a diverse range of antioxidants and other essential nutrients.

Green Tea

Green tea is not only a popular beverage but also a rich source of antioxidants called catechins. Catechins have been shown to have powerful antioxidant and anti-inflammatory properties. Regular consumption of green tea has been linked to a reduced risk of heart disease, certain types of cancer, and improved brain function. To maximize the antioxidant benefits, opt for high-quality loose-leaf green tea and steep it for the recommended time.

Turmeric

Turmeric is a spice commonly used in Indian cuisine and is known for its vibrant yellow color. It contains a compound called curcumin, which is a potent antioxidant and has strong anti-inflammatory properties. Curcumin has been studied for its potential benefits in reducing the risk of chronic diseases such as heart disease, cancer, and Alzheimer's disease. To enhance the absorption of curcumin, it is recommended to consume turmeric with black pepper or in combination with healthy fats.

Beans and Legumes

Beans and legumes, such as kidney beans, black beans, lentils, and chickpeas, are not only an excellent source of plant-based protein and fiber but also contain a variety of antioxidants. These antioxidant-rich foods are particularly high in flavonoids, which have been shown to have anti-inflammatory and anticancer properties. Including a variety of beans and legumes in your diet can provide a significant antioxidant boost while promoting overall health and well-being.

Conclusion

Incorporating antioxidant-rich foods into your daily diet is a simple and effective way to enhance your overall health and well-being. By consuming a variety of these foods, such as berries, dark chocolate, green leafy vegetables, nuts and seeds, colorful vegetables and fruits, green tea, turmeric, and beans and legumes, you can ensure a diverse range of antioxidants that provide numerous health benefits. Remember to aim for a balanced and varied diet to maximize your antioxidant intake and support optimal health.

Incorporating Antioxidant Rich Foods into Your Meals

Incorporating antioxidant-rich foods into your meals is a simple and effective way to boost your overall health and well-being. Antioxidants play a crucial role in protecting your body against harmful free radicals, which can cause oxidative stress and damage to your cells. By including a variety of antioxidant-rich foods in your diet, you can help reduce the risk of chronic diseases, improve your immune system, and promote healthy aging.

When it comes to incorporating antioxidant-rich foods into your meals, the key is to focus on variety and balance. Different foods contain different types and amounts of antioxidants, so it's important to include a wide range of fruits, vegetables, whole grains, nuts, and seeds in your diet. Here are some practical tips and examples to help you get started:

·

Start your day with a nutritious breakfast: Kickstart your morning with a breakfast that includes antioxidant-rich foods. For example, you can enjoy a bowl of oatmeal topped with fresh berries like blueberries, strawberries, or raspberries. These berries are packed with antioxidants such as anthocyanins, which have been shown to have anti-inflammatory and anti-cancer properties.

·

·

Snack on antioxidant-rich fruits: Instead of reaching for processed snacks, opt for antioxidant-rich fruits as a healthy and satisfying snack. Apples, oranges, grapes, and cherries are all excellent choices. You can also create a colorful fruit salad by combining different fruits to maximize your antioxidant intake.

·

·

Add leafy greens to your meals: Leafy greens like spinach, kale, and Swiss chard are not only rich in antioxidants but also provide a wide range of other essential nutrients. Incorporate them into your meals by adding them to salads, stir-fries, or smoothies. For example, you can make a nutrient-packed salad with spinach, mixed berries, walnuts, and a drizzle of olive oil.

·

·

Include colorful vegetables in your dishes: Colorful vegetables such as bell peppers, tomatoes, carrots, and sweet potatoes are not only visually appealing but also packed with antioxidants. Roast them in the oven with a sprinkle of herbs and spices for a flavorful side dish or add them to soups and stews for an extra nutritional boost.

·

·

Experiment with herbs and spices: Many herbs and spices are known for their antioxidant properties. Turmeric, ginger, cinnamon, and oregano are just a few examples. Incorporate these flavorful ingredients into your cooking to enhance the antioxidant content of your meals. For instance, you can add turmeric and ginger to a stir-fry or sprinkle cinnamon on your morning oatmeal.

.

.

Include whole grains in your diet: Whole grains like quinoa, brown rice, and whole wheat bread are not only a great source of fiber but also contain antioxidants. Swap refined grains for whole grains in your meals to increase your antioxidant intake. For example, you can enjoy a quinoa salad with roasted vegetables or have a whole grain sandwich with avocado and tomato.

.

.

Don't forget about nuts and seeds: Nuts and seeds are not only a convenient and portable snack but also provide a good amount of antioxidants. Almonds, walnuts, flaxseeds, and chia seeds are all excellent choices. Sprinkle them on top of your salads, yogurt, or smoothies for an added crunch and nutritional boost.

.

.

Enjoy a cup of antioxidant-rich tea: Green tea, black tea, and herbal teas like chamomile and rooibos are all rich in antioxidants. Replace sugary beverages with a cup of antioxidant-rich tea to hydrate your body and reap the benefits of these powerful compounds.

.

Remember, incorporating antioxidant-rich foods into your meals doesn't have to be complicated. By making small changes and being mindful of your food choices, you can easily increase your antioxidant intake and support your overall health. Aim for a colorful and varied plate, and don't be afraid to try new recipes and flavors. Your body will thank you for nourishing it with these nutrient-dense foods.

Recipes Featuring Antioxidant Rich Ingredients

Antioxidants play a crucial role in protecting our bodies from harmful free radicals and reducing the risk of chronic diseases. Incorporating antioxidant-rich foods into our diet is essential for maintaining optimal health. In this section, we will explore some delicious recipes that feature ingredients packed with antioxidants.

Blueberry Spinach Smoothie

Ingredients:

- 1 cup fresh or frozen blueberries
- 1 cup spinach leaves
- 1 ripe banana
- 1 cup almond milk (or any milk of your choice)
- 1 tablespoon chia seeds
- 1 tablespoon honey (optional)

Instructions:

- In a blender, combine the blueberries, spinach, banana, almond milk, chia seeds, and honey (if desired).
- Blend until smooth and creamy.
- Pour into a glass and enjoy this refreshing and antioxidant-rich smoothie.

Blueberries are known for their high antioxidant content, particularly anthocyanins, which give them their vibrant color. Spinach is also a great source of antioxidants, including vitamins A and C. This smoothie is not only delicious but also a fantastic way to start your day with a boost of antioxidants.

Quinoa Salad with Mixed Berries

Ingredients:

- 1 cup cooked quinoa
- 1 cup mixed berries (such as strawberries, raspberries, and blackberries)
- 1/4 cup chopped fresh mint leaves

- 1/4 cup crumbled feta cheese
- 2 tablespoons chopped almonds
- 2 tablespoons extra-virgin olive oil
- 1 tablespoon balsamic vinegar
- Salt and pepper to taste

Instructions:

- In a large bowl, combine the cooked quinoa, mixed berries, mint leaves, feta cheese, and chopped almonds.
- In a separate small bowl, whisk together the olive oil, balsamic vinegar, salt, and pepper.
- Drizzle the dressing over the quinoa salad and toss gently to combine.
- Serve chilled and enjoy this nutritious and antioxidant-packed salad.

Berries are well-known for their antioxidant properties, and this salad combines a variety of them to create a burst of flavors. Quinoa adds a protein punch, while the fresh mint leaves and feta cheese provide a refreshing and tangy twist.

Roasted Vegetable Medley

Ingredients:

- 1 cup cherry tomatoes
- 1 cup chopped bell peppers (assorted colors)
- 1 cup chopped zucchini
- 1 cup chopped eggplant
- 1 tablespoon extra-virgin olive oil
- 1 teaspoon dried herbs (such as thyme or rosemary)
- Salt and pepper to taste

Instructions:

- Preheat the oven to 400°F (200°C).
- In a large baking dish, combine the cherry tomatoes, bell peppers, zucchini, and eggplant.
- Drizzle the vegetables with olive oil and sprinkle with dried herbs, salt, and pepper.
- Toss the vegetables to coat them evenly with the oil

and seasonings.

- Roast in the preheated oven for 25-30 minutes or until the vegetables are tender and slightly caramelized.
- Remove from the oven and let cool slightly before serving.

This roasted vegetable medley is not only a feast for the eyes but also a powerhouse of antioxidants. Tomatoes, bell peppers, zucchini, and eggplant are all rich in antioxidants, vitamins, and minerals. Enjoy this colorful and flavorful dish as a side or as a main course with some whole grains or lean protein.

Dark Chocolate Berry Bark

Ingredients:

- 1 cup dark chocolate chips (at least 70% cocoa)
- 1/2 cup mixed berries (such as blueberries, raspberries, and dried cranberries)
- 2 tablespoons chopped pistachios (optional)

Instructions:

- Line a baking sheet with parchment paper.
- Melt the dark chocolate chips in a microwave-safe bowl in 30-second intervals, stirring in between, until smooth and melted.
- Pour the melted chocolate onto the prepared baking sheet and spread it evenly with a spatula.
- Sprinkle the mixed berries and chopped pistachios (if using) over the melted chocolate, pressing them gently into the surface.
- Place the baking sheet in the refrigerator for about 30 minutes or until the chocolate hardens.
- Once hardened, break the bark into small pieces and store in an airtight container.

Dark chocolate is a rich source of antioxidants, particularly flavonoids, which have been associated with various health benefits. This dark chocolate berry bark is a delightful and guilt-free treat that combines the antioxidant power of dark chocolate with the vibrant flavors of mixed berries and the crunch of pistachios.

These recipes are just a glimpse of the many ways you can incorporate antioxidant-rich ingredients into your meals. Get creative in the kitchen and explore different combinations to enjoy the benefits of these nutrient-packed foods. Remember, a diet rich in antioxidants is a key component of a healthy and balanced lifestyle.

SUPERFOODS

What Makes a Food a Superfood?

Superfoods have gained significant popularity in recent years due to their exceptional nutritional value and potential health benefits. But what exactly makes a food a superfood? Is it just a marketing term, or is there scientific evidence to support their claims?

In simple terms, superfoods are nutrient powerhouses that are packed with a high concentration of vitamins, minerals, antioxidants, and other beneficial compounds. These foods go above and beyond the basic nutritional requirements and offer additional health-promoting properties. They are often associated with reducing the risk of chronic diseases, boosting the immune system, improving cognitive function, and promoting overall well-being.

One of the key characteristics of superfoods is their high nutrient density. Nutrient density refers to the amount of essential nutrients per calorie in a food. Superfoods are typically low in calories but rich in essential vitamins, minerals, and antioxidants. This means that even small portions of these foods can provide a significant amount of nutrients, making them an excellent choice for those looking to maximize their nutritional intake.

Another important aspect of superfoods is their unique composition of bioactive compounds. These compounds are naturally occurring substances found in plants that have been shown to have positive effects on human health. For example, berries such as blueberries and strawberries are rich in anthocyanins, which have been linked to improved brain function and reduced risk of heart disease. Turmeric, a spice commonly used in Indian cuisine, contains curcumin, a powerful anti-inflammatory compound with potential cancer-fighting properties.

Superfoods also tend to be rich in antioxidants. Antioxidants are compounds that help protect our cells from damage caused by harmful molecules called free radicals. Free radicals can contribute to the development of chronic diseases such as cancer, heart disease, and aging. By consuming foods high in antioxidants, we can help neutralize these free radicals and reduce the risk of oxidative stress.

Examples of superfoods include:

.

Berries: Blueberries, strawberries, raspberries, and blackberries are all packed with antioxidants, fiber, and vitamins.

.

.

Leafy greens: Spinach, kale, Swiss chard, and collard greens are nutrient powerhouses, providing an abundance of vitamins A, C, and K, as well as minerals like iron and calcium.

.

.

Nuts and seeds: Almonds, walnuts, chia seeds, and flaxseeds are excellent sources of healthy fats, fiber, and essential minerals.

-

-

Fish: Fatty fish such as salmon, mackerel, and sardines are rich in omega-3 fatty acids, which have been shown to support heart health and brain function.

-

-

Legumes: Beans, lentils, and chickpeas are high in protein, fiber, and various vitamins and minerals.

-

-

Whole grains: Quinoa, brown rice, oats, and barley are nutrient-dense grains that provide fiber, B vitamins, and minerals.

-

-

Cruciferous vegetables: Broccoli, cauliflower, Brussels sprouts, and cabbage are packed with vitamins, minerals, and cancer-fighting compounds.

-

-

Green tea: Known for its high concentration of antioxidants, green tea has been associated with numerous health benefits, including improved brain function and a reduced risk of heart disease.

-

It's important to note that while superfoods can be a valuable addition to a healthy diet, they should not be considered a magical solution or a replacement for a balanced eating plan. Variety and moderation are key when it comes to nutrition. Incorporating a wide range of nutrient-rich foods into your diet is the best way to ensure you're getting all the essential nutrients your body needs.

In the next section, we will explore different types of superfoods in more detail, highlighting their specific health benefits and ways to incorporate them into your daily diet.

Exploring Different Types of Superfoods

Superfoods have gained popularity in recent years due to their exceptional nutritional value and health benefits. These foods are packed with a wide range of essential nutrients, including vitamins, minerals, antioxidants, and phytochemicals. Incorporating superfoods into your diet can help boost your immune system, improve digestion, enhance brain function, and promote overall well-being. In this section, we will explore different types of superfoods and their unique properties.

Berries

Berries are a delicious and nutritious addition to any diet. They are rich in antioxidants, which help protect the body against free radicals and reduce the risk of chronic diseases such as heart disease and cancer. Some popular berries include blueberries, strawberries, raspberries, and blackberries. Blueberries, in particular, are known for their high levels of anthocyanins, which have been linked to improved brain function and memory. You can enjoy berries on their own, add them to smoothies, or sprinkle them over yogurt or oatmeal for a burst of flavor and nutrients.

Leafy Greens

Leafy greens such as spinach, kale, and Swiss chard are nutritional powerhouses. They are packed with vitamins A, C, and K, as well as folate, iron, and fiber. These greens are low in calories and high in antioxidants, making them an excellent choice for weight management and overall health. Spinach, for example, is rich in lutein and zeaxanthin, which promote eye health and reduce the risk of age-related macular degeneration. You can incorporate leafy greens into your diet by adding them to salads, stir-fries, or smoothies.

Cruciferous Vegetables

Cruciferous vegetables belong to the Brassicaceae family and include broccoli, cauliflower, Brussels sprouts, and cabbage. These vegetables are known for their cancer-fighting properties due to their high content of glucosinolates, which are converted into compounds that help detoxify the body and reduce inflammation. Broccoli, in particular, is a great source of vitamin C, fiber, and folate. You can enjoy cruciferous vegetables by steaming, roasting, or sautéing them as a side dish or adding them to stir-fries and soups.

Nuts and Seeds

Nuts and seeds are nutrient-dense foods that provide a wide range of health benefits. They are rich in healthy fats, protein, fiber, vitamins, and minerals. Almonds, for example, are a great source of vitamin E, magnesium, and calcium. Walnuts are high in omega-3 fatty acids, which are essential for brain health. Chia seeds are packed with fiber and omega-3 fatty acids, while flaxseeds are rich in lignans, which have antioxidant and anti-inflammatory properties. You can enjoy nuts and seeds as a snack, sprinkle them over salads or yogurt, or use them in baking and cooking.

Fish

Fatty fish such as salmon, mackerel, and sardines are excellent sources of omega-3 fatty acids, which are essential for heart health and brain function. Omega-3 fatty acids have been shown to reduce inflammation, lower blood pressure, and improve cholesterol levels. These fish are also rich in high-quality protein, vitamins D and B12, and minerals such as selenium and iodine. Aim to include fatty fish in your diet at least twice a week by grilling, baking, or poaching them.

Legumes

Legumes, including beans, lentils, and chickpeas, are a great source of plant-based protein, fiber, and complex carbohydrates. They are also rich in vitamins and minerals such as folate, iron, and potassium. Legumes have been associated with a reduced risk of heart disease, diabetes, and certain types of cancer. Chickpeas, for example, are high in fiber and protein, making them a great addition to salads, soups, and stews. Lentils are rich in folate and iron, while black beans are packed with antioxidants and fiber.

Whole Grains

Whole grains such as quinoa, brown rice, oats, and whole wheat are an essential part of a nutrient-rich diet. They are rich in fiber, vitamins, minerals, and antioxidants. Whole grains have been linked to a reduced risk of heart disease, type 2 diabetes, and obesity. Quinoa, for example, is a complete protein and a good source of iron and magnesium. Brown rice is high in fiber and B vitamins, while oats are rich in beta-glucan, a type of soluble fiber that helps lower cholesterol levels. Incorporate whole grains into your meals by replacing refined grains with whole grain options.

Conclusion

Superfoods offer a wide range of health benefits and can be easily incorporated into your daily diet. Berries, leafy greens, cruciferous vegetables, nuts and seeds, fish, legumes, and whole grains are just a few examples of superfoods that can help optimize your nutrition and promote overall well-being. Experiment with different types of superfoods and find creative ways to include them in your meals. By incorporating these nutrient-rich foods into your diet, you can take a significant step towards achieving optimal health and vitality.

Incorporating Superfoods into Your Daily Diet

Superfoods have gained popularity in recent years due to their exceptional nutritional value and health benefits. These foods are packed with essential vitamins, minerals, antioxidants, and other beneficial compounds that can support overall well-being and help prevent chronic diseases. Incorporating superfoods into your daily diet is a fantastic way to enhance your nutrient intake and optimize your health. In this section, we will explore various strategies and practical tips to seamlessly integrate these nutritional powerhouses into your meals.

One of the simplest ways to incorporate superfoods into your daily diet is by adding them to your favorite recipes. For example, you can sprinkle chia seeds or flaxseeds onto your morning oatmeal or yogurt for an extra boost of omega-3 fatty acids and fiber. These tiny seeds are also versatile and can be used as an egg substitute in baking or as a thickening agent in smoothies.

Another superfood that can easily be incorporated into your diet is spinach. This leafy green is rich in vitamins A, C, and K, as well as iron and calcium. You can add spinach to your salads, stir-fries, omelets, or even blend it into your smoothies for a nutrient-packed green boost. Similarly, kale, another nutrient-dense leafy green, can be sautéed, roasted, or used as a base for salads.

Berries, such as blueberries, strawberries, and raspberries, are excellent sources of antioxidants and can be enjoyed in various ways. You can add them to your morning cereal, blend them into smoothies, or simply enjoy them as a refreshing snack. Additionally, you can experiment with different types of berries to create delicious and nutritious desserts like berry crumbles or compotes.

Quinoa, a gluten-free grain, is considered a superfood due to its high protein content and essential amino acids. It can be used as a substitute for rice or pasta in many dishes. Quinoa salads, stir-fries, and pilafs are popular options that allow you to incorporate this superfood into your meals while enjoying its nutty flavor and satisfying texture.

Avocado, often referred to as a superfood, is a rich source of healthy fats, fiber, and various vitamins and minerals. You can spread avocado on toast, add it to salads, or use it as a creamy base for dressings and sauces. Additionally, you can use avocado as a substitute for butter or oil in baking recipes to reduce the saturated fat content while adding a unique creaminess.

Turmeric, a vibrant yellow spice, contains a compound called curcumin, which has potent anti-inflammatory properties. You can incorporate turmeric into your diet by adding it to curries, soups, or roasted vegetables. Golden milk, a warm beverage made with turmeric, milk, and spices, is also a popular way to enjoy the benefits of this superfood.

Incorporating superfoods into your daily diet doesn't have to be complicated or time-consuming. You can start by making small changes and gradually increase your intake over time. For example, you can swap your regular white rice with nutrient-rich quinoa or replace your usual cooking oil with extra virgin olive oil, which is known for its heart-healthy properties.

Another effective strategy is to plan your meals around superfoods. Include a variety of superfoods in your weekly meal plan to ensure you're getting a wide range of nutrients. For instance, you can plan to have a salmon salad with mixed greens, avocado, and berries for lunch, followed by a dinner of roasted sweet potatoes, broccoli, and grilled chicken seasoned with turmeric.

Smoothies are also an excellent way to incorporate multiple superfoods into one delicious and convenient meal. You can blend together spinach, berries, chia seeds, and a scoop of protein powder for a nutrient-packed breakfast or post-workout snack. Experiment with different combinations to find your favorite superfood smoothie recipe.

Lastly, don't forget to read food labels and choose packaged products that contain superfoods. Look for snacks or granola bars that include ingredients like nuts, seeds, dark chocolate, or dried fruits. However, it's important to note that whole foods are generally a better choice than processed foods, as they provide a more significant nutritional punch.

Incorporating superfoods into your daily diet is an exciting and rewarding journey towards optimal health. By making simple swaps, planning your meals strategically, and experimenting with new recipes, you can enjoy the benefits of these nutrient-rich foods while savoring delicious flavors and textures. Remember, small changes can lead to significant improvements in your overall well-being. So, start incorporating superfoods into your daily diet today and reap the rewards of a nutrient-rich lifestyle.

Superfood Recipes for Optimal Nutrition

Superfoods are nutrient powerhouses that provide a wide range of essential vitamins, minerals, and antioxidants. Incorporating these foods into your diet can help boost your overall health and well-being. In this section, we will explore some delicious and nutritious superfood recipes that you can easily incorporate into your daily meals.

Recipe 1: Quinoa and Kale Salad

Ingredients:

- 1 cup cooked quinoa
- 2 cups chopped kale
- 1 cup cherry tomatoes, halved
- 1/2 cup diced cucumber
- 1/4 cup chopped red onion
- 1/4 cup crumbled feta cheese
- 2 tablespoons extra virgin olive oil
- 1 tablespoon lemon juice
- Salt and pepper to taste

Instructions:

- In a large bowl, combine the cooked quinoa, chopped kale, cherry tomatoes, cucumber, red onion, and feta cheese.
- In a small bowl, whisk together the olive oil, lemon juice, salt, and pepper.
- Pour the dressing over the salad and toss well to combine.
- Let the salad sit for at least 10 minutes to allow the flavors to meld together.
- Serve as a side dish or add grilled chicken or tofu for a complete meal.

Recipe 2: Berry Chia Pudding

Ingredients:

- 1/4 cup chia seeds
- 1 cup unsweetened almond milk
- 1/2 cup mixed berries (such as blueberries, raspberries, and strawberries)
- 1 tablespoon honey or maple syrup (optional)
- 1/4 teaspoon vanilla extract

Instructions:

- In a jar or bowl, combine the chia seeds and almond milk. Stir well to ensure the chia seeds are evenly distributed.
- Let the mixture sit for 5 minutes, then stir again to prevent clumping.
- Cover the jar or bowl and refrigerate overnight or for at least 4 hours.
- In the morning or when ready to serve, give the chia pudding a good stir to break up any clumps.
- Top with mixed berries and drizzle with honey or maple syrup, if desired.
- Add a splash of vanilla extract for extra flavor.
- Enjoy as a healthy breakfast or snack option.

Recipe 3: Salmon and Avocado Sushi Rolls

Ingredients:

- 2 cups cooked sushi rice
- 4 nori seaweed sheets
- 1/2 pound fresh salmon, thinly sliced
- 1 avocado, sliced
- 1/4 cup low-sodium soy sauce
- Wasabi and pickled ginger for serving (optional)

Instructions:

- Lay a bamboo sushi mat on a clean surface and place a nori sheet on top.
- Wet your hands with water to prevent sticking, then spread a thin layer of sushi rice evenly over the nori sheet, leaving a 1-inch border at the top.
- Lay slices of salmon and avocado in a line across the center of the rice.

. Using the bamboo mat, roll the sushi tightly, applying gentle pressure to ensure it holds together.

. Repeat the process with the remaining nori sheets and ingredients.

. Use a sharp knife to slice each roll into bite-sized pieces.

. Serve with low-sodium soy sauce, wasabi, and pickled ginger, if desired.

Recipe 4: Spinach and Blueberry Smoothie

Ingredients:

- 2 cups fresh spinach
- 1 cup frozen blueberries
- 1 ripe banana
- 1 cup unsweetened almond milk
- 1 tablespoon almond butter
- 1 tablespoon honey or maple syrup (optional)
- Ice cubes (optional)

Instructions:

. In a blender, combine the spinach, blueberries, banana, almond milk, almond butter, and honey or maple syrup.

. Blend until smooth and creamy.

. If desired, add a few ice cubes and blend again until well combined.

. Pour into a glass and enjoy as a refreshing and nutrient-rich smoothie.

Recipe 5: Turmeric Roasted Cauliflower

Ingredients:

- 1 head cauliflower, cut into florets
- 2 tablespoons olive oil
- 1 teaspoon ground turmeric
- 1/2 teaspoon ground cumin
- 1/2 teaspoon paprika
- Salt and pepper to taste

Instructions:

- Preheat the oven to 400°F (200°C).
- In a large bowl, combine the cauliflower florets, olive oil, turmeric, cumin, paprika, salt, and pepper. Toss well to coat the cauliflower evenly.
- Spread the cauliflower in a single layer on a baking sheet.
- Roast in the preheated oven for 25-30 minutes, or until the cauliflower is tender and golden brown.
- Serve as a side dish or add to salads, grain bowls, or wraps for an extra boost of flavor and nutrition.

These superfood recipes are just a starting point for incorporating nutrient-rich foods into your diet. Feel free to experiment with different ingredients and flavors to create your own delicious and nutritious meals. Remember, the key is to choose a variety of superfoods to ensure you're getting a wide range of essential nutrients for optimal health and well-being.

FRUITS AND VEGETABLES

The Nutritional Powerhouses

Fruits and vegetables are often referred to as the nutritional powerhouses of our diet. Packed with essential vitamins, minerals, fiber, and antioxidants, these plant-based foods offer a wide range of health benefits. Incorporating a variety of fruits and vegetables into your daily meals can help support overall health and well-being.

The Importance of Fruits and Vegetables

Fruits and vegetables are essential for maintaining a balanced and nutrient-rich diet. They provide a wide array of vitamins and minerals that are crucial for various bodily functions. For example, vitamin C found in citrus fruits helps boost the immune system and promotes healthy skin. Leafy green vegetables like spinach and kale are rich in vitamin K, which plays a vital role in blood clotting and bone health.

In addition to vitamins and minerals, fruits and vegetables are also excellent sources of dietary fiber. Fiber aids in digestion, helps regulate blood sugar levels, and promotes a feeling of fullness, which can aid in weight management. By including a variety of fruits and vegetables in your meals, you can ensure you're getting an adequate amount of fiber to support a healthy digestive system.

Nutrient Content of Fruits and Vegetables

Different fruits and vegetables offer unique nutritional profiles. Here are some examples of the nutrient content of commonly consumed fruits and vegetables:

- **Berries**: Berries such as strawberries, blueberries, and raspberries are rich in antioxidants, which help protect the body against oxidative stress and inflammation. They are also a good source of vitamin C and dietary fiber.

-
- **Leafy Greens**: Leafy greens like spinach, kale, and Swiss chard are packed with vitamins A, C, and K, as well as folate and iron. These greens are also low in calories and high in fiber, making them an excellent choice for weight management.

-
- **Citrus Fruits**: Citrus fruits like oranges, grapefruits, and lemons are known for their high vitamin C content. They also provide potassium, folate, and fiber. Citrus fruits are refreshing and can be enjoyed as a snack or added to salads and smoothies.

-
- **Cruciferous Vegetables**: Cruciferous vegetables such as broccoli, cauliflower, and Brussels sprouts are rich in vitamins C, K, and folate. They also contain compounds called glucosinolates, which have been linked to a reduced risk of certain types of

cancer.

.

.

Root Vegetables: Root vegetables like carrots, sweet potatoes, and beets are excellent sources of beta-carotene, which the body converts into vitamin A. They also provide fiber and other essential nutrients.

.

.

Tomatoes: Tomatoes are rich in lycopene, a powerful antioxidant that has been associated with a reduced risk of heart disease and certain types of cancer. They are also a good source of vitamins A and C.

.

These are just a few examples of the nutrient content found in fruits and vegetables. By incorporating a variety of these foods into your diet, you can ensure you're getting a wide range of essential vitamins, minerals, and antioxidants.

Health Benefits of Fruits and Vegetables

Including ample amounts of fruits and vegetables in your diet can have numerous health benefits. Here are some of the key advantages:

.

Heart Health: The high fiber content in fruits and vegetables, along with their low-calorie nature, can help maintain healthy cholesterol levels and reduce the risk of heart disease.

.

.

Weight Management: Fruits and vegetables are low in calories and high in fiber, making them an excellent choice for weight management. They provide essential nutrients while helping you feel full and satisfied.

.

.

Digestive Health: The fiber content in fruits and vegetables promotes healthy digestion and prevents constipation. It also supports the growth of beneficial gut bacteria, which is essential for overall gut health.

.

.

Cancer Prevention: Many fruits and vegetables contain antioxidants and phytochemicals that have been linked to a reduced risk of certain types of cancer. These compounds help protect cells from damage and inhibit the growth of cancer cells.

.

.

Eye Health: Fruits and vegetables rich in vitamins A and C, such as carrots and bell peppers, are beneficial for eye health. They help protect against age-related macular degeneration and maintain good vision.

.

.

Skin Health: The vitamins and antioxidants found in fruits and vegetables contribute to healthy skin. They help protect against oxidative stress, promote collagen production, and maintain a youthful appearance.

.

Incorporating Fruits and Vegetables into Your Diet

To reap the benefits of fruits and vegetables, it's important to incorporate them into your daily meals. Here are some tips for increasing your intake:

.

Variety: Aim to include a variety of fruits and vegetables in your diet to ensure you're getting a wide range of nutrients. Experiment with different colors, textures, and flavors to keep your meals interesting.

.

.

Fresh and Seasonal: Choose fresh, locally grown produce whenever possible. Seasonal fruits and vegetables are often more flavorful and nutrient-dense. Visit farmers' markets or consider growing your own garden to access fresh produce.

·

·

Snacks and Side Dishes: Incorporate fruits and vegetables into your snacks and side dishes. Cut up fresh fruits for a refreshing snack or add vegetables to salads, stir-fries, and soups.

·

·

Smoothies and Juices: Blend fruits and vegetables into smoothies or make fresh juices to increase your intake. These can be a convenient way to consume a variety of nutrients in one serving.

·

·

Meal Planning: Plan your meals in advance and include fruits and vegetables in each meal. This will ensure that you have a balanced and nutrient-rich diet throughout the week.

·

Remember, the key is to make fruits and vegetables a regular part of your diet. By doing so, you'll be nourishing your body with essential nutrients and reaping the numerous health benefits they offer.

The Nutritional Powerhouses

Fruits and vegetables are often referred to as the nutritional powerhouses of our diet, and for good reason. Packed with essential vitamins, minerals, fiber, and antioxidants, these plant-based foods provide a wide range of health benefits and play a crucial role in maintaining optimal health.

The Importance of Fruits and Vegetables

Fruits and vegetables are essential for a well-balanced and nutrient-rich diet. They are low in calories and high in nutrients, making them an excellent choice for weight management and overall health. These plant-based foods are rich in vitamins A, C, and E, as well as minerals like potassium and magnesium. They also contain phytochemicals, which are natural compounds that have been shown to have numerous health benefits, including reducing the risk of chronic diseases such as heart disease, cancer, and diabetes.

Nutrient Content of Fruits and Vegetables

Different fruits and vegetables offer a variety of nutrients, so it's important to include a wide range of colors and types in your diet. Here are some examples of the nutrient content of popular fruits and vegetables:

-

Leafy Greens: Spinach, kale, and Swiss chard are excellent sources of vitamins A, C, and K, as well as folate and iron. These greens are also rich in antioxidants, which help protect the body against oxidative stress and inflammation.

-

-

Citrus Fruits: Oranges, grapefruits, and lemons are packed with vitamin C, which is essential for a healthy immune system and collagen production. They also provide dietary fiber and various antioxidants that support overall health.

-

-

Berries: Blueberries, strawberries, and raspberries are known for their high antioxidant content. They are also a good source of fiber, vitamins C and K, and manganese. Berries have been linked to improved brain health, heart health, and reduced inflammation.

-

-

Cruciferous Vegetables: Broccoli, cauliflower, and Brussels sprouts are part of the cruciferous vegetable family, known for their cancer-fighting properties. They are rich in vitamins C and K, folate, and fiber. These vegetables also contain sulforaphane, a compound that has been shown to have anti-inflammatory and antioxidant effects.

•

•

Root Vegetables: Carrots, sweet potatoes, and beets are packed with vitamins A and C, as well as fiber and potassium. These vegetables are known for their vibrant colors and provide a range of health benefits, including improved eye health and enhanced digestion.

•

•

Tomatoes: Tomatoes are a great source of vitamins A and C, as well as lycopene, a powerful antioxidant. Lycopene has been associated with a reduced risk of certain types of cancer, particularly prostate cancer. Tomatoes also provide potassium and fiber.

•

•

Avocado: Avocado is a unique fruit that is rich in healthy fats, particularly monounsaturated fats. It also provides vitamins K, C, E, and B-6, as well as folate and potassium. Avocado is known for its heart-healthy properties and its ability to enhance nutrient absorption from other foods.

•

Incorporating Fruits and Vegetables into Your Diet

To reap the full benefits of fruits and vegetables, it's important to incorporate them into your daily meals and snacks. Here are some practical tips for increasing your intake:

•

Variety is key: Aim to include a variety of fruits and vegetables in your diet to ensure you're getting a wide range of nutrients. Experiment with different colors, textures, and flavors to keep your meals interesting.

•

•

Fresh is best: Whenever possible, choose fresh fruits and vegetables over canned or processed options. Fresh produce tends to have higher nutrient content and better flavor. If fresh produce is not available, frozen fruits and vegetables can be a convenient and nutritious alternative.

-

-

Add them to every meal: Make it a habit to include fruits and vegetables in every meal. Add berries to your breakfast cereal, include a side salad with lunch and dinner, and incorporate vegetables into your main dishes. You can also snack on raw vegetables or enjoy a piece of fruit as a healthy dessert.

-

-

Get creative: Experiment with different cooking methods and recipes to make fruits and vegetables more appealing. Roasting, grilling, and sautéing can enhance the flavors and textures of these foods. You can also try blending fruits into smoothies or making vegetable-based soups and stews.

-

-

Grow your own: If you have the space and resources, consider starting a small garden to grow your own fruits and vegetables. This can be a rewarding and cost-effective way to ensure a fresh supply of nutritious produce.

-

Remember, the key is to make fruits and vegetables a central part of your diet. By incorporating these nutritional powerhouses into your meals and snacks, you'll be well on your way to achieving optimal health and vitality.

Creative Ways to Enjoy Fruits and Vegetables

Fruits and vegetables are the nutritional powerhouses of our diet. They are packed with essential vitamins, minerals, fiber, and antioxidants that promote good health and protect against chronic diseases. While it's important to include a variety of fruits and vegetables in our diet, it can sometimes be challenging to find creative ways to enjoy them. In this section, we will explore some innovative and delicious ways to incorporate more fruits and vegetables into your meals.

1. Smoothies and Juices

Smoothies and juices are a fantastic way to enjoy a variety of fruits and vegetables in one refreshing drink. You can experiment with different combinations to create your own unique flavors. For example, a green smoothie made with spinach, kale, banana, and almond milk is not only nutritious but also delicious. You can also add fruits like berries, mangoes, or pineapples to enhance the taste. Similarly, fresh vegetable juices like carrot, beetroot, or cucumber can be mixed with fruits like oranges or apples for a vibrant and nutrient-rich beverage.

2. Salads with a Twist

Salads don't have to be boring! Get creative with your salad ingredients to make them more exciting and flavorful. Add a variety of colorful fruits like strawberries, blueberries, or pomegranate seeds to your green salads for a burst of sweetness. You can also incorporate vegetables like roasted beets, grilled zucchini, or caramelized onions to add depth and texture. Don't forget to experiment with different dressings like citrus vinaigrette, honey mustard, or tahini-based dressings to elevate the flavors even more.

3. Veggie Noodles

Replace traditional pasta with veggie noodles for a healthier and lighter alternative. You can make noodles from zucchini, carrots, sweet potatoes, or butternut squash using a spiralizer or a vegetable peeler. These veggie noodles can be sautéed, stir-fried, or even enjoyed raw in salads. Top them with your favorite sauces, such as marinara, pesto, or peanut sauce, and add some protein like grilled chicken or tofu for a complete and satisfying meal.

4. Stuffed Vegetables

Get creative with stuffed vegetables to make a nutritious and visually appealing dish. Bell peppers, zucchini, tomatoes, and mushrooms are great options for stuffing. You can fill them with a variety of ingredients like quinoa, lentils, couscous, or even a mixture of sautéed vegetables and cheese. Bake or grill the stuffed vegetables until they are tender and the flavors meld together. This is a great way to enjoy a balanced meal with a variety of nutrients.

5. Fruit Salsa and Sides

Fruit salsa is a refreshing and versatile accompaniment to many dishes. Combine diced fruits like mangoes, pineapples, strawberries, or peaches with herbs like cilantro or mint, and add a squeeze of lime juice for a burst of flavor. Fruit salsa can be served as a topping for grilled chicken or fish, as a dip with whole-grain tortilla chips, or even as a side dish to complement a savory meal. It adds a delightful sweetness and tanginess to any dish.

6. Roasted Vegetables

Roasting vegetables brings out their natural sweetness and enhances their flavors. You can roast a variety of vegetables like broccoli, cauliflower, Brussels sprouts, sweet potatoes, or bell peppers. Toss them with olive oil, salt, and your favorite herbs and spices, then roast them in the oven until they are caramelized and tender. Roasted vegetables can be enjoyed as a side dish, added to salads, or even used as a topping for pizzas or sandwiches.

7. Fruit and Vegetable Skewers

Skewers are a fun and interactive way to enjoy fruits and vegetables. Thread a variety of colorful fruits like melons, grapes, kiwis, and berries onto skewers for a refreshing and healthy dessert option. You can also make savory skewers with vegetables like cherry tomatoes, bell peppers, mushrooms, and onions. Grill or bake the skewers until the vegetables are tender and slightly charred. Serve them as an appetizer or as a side dish with your favorite dipping sauce.

8. Veggie Burgers and Patties

Replace meat patties with veggie burgers or patties for a nutritious and plant-based alternative. You can make patties using ingredients like black beans, chickpeas, lentils, or quinoa. Add a variety of vegetables, herbs, and spices to enhance the flavors. Grill or bake the patties until they are crispy on the outside and tender on the inside. Serve them on whole-grain buns with your favorite toppings and condiments for a satisfying and nutrient-rich meal.

9. Fruit and Vegetable Desserts

Who said desserts can't be healthy? Get creative with fruits and vegetables to make delicious and guilt-free desserts. For example, you can make a fruit salad with a variety of seasonal fruits and top it with a dollop of Greek yogurt and a sprinkle of nuts for added crunch. You can also bake fruit crisps or cobblers using fruits like apples, berries, or peaches, and top them with a whole-grain crumble. Another option is to make vegetable-based desserts like carrot cake, zucchini bread, or sweet potato brownies for a nutrient-rich treat.

10. Fruity and Veggie Popsicles

Beat the heat with homemade fruity and veggie popsicles. Blend a variety of fruits like watermelon, berries, or mangoes with a little bit of water or coconut water, and pour the mixture into popsicle molds. You can also add pureed vegetables like spinach, cucumber, or beets for an extra nutritional boost. Freeze the popsicles until they are solid, and enjoy a refreshing and healthy treat on a hot day.

Remember, the key to enjoying fruits and vegetables is to experiment with different flavors, textures, and cooking methods. Don't be afraid to try new recipes and combinations. By getting creative with your fruits and vegetables, you can make healthy eating exciting and enjoyable for the whole family.

Seasonal Eating

Seasonal eating is a concept that involves consuming foods that are naturally grown and harvested during specific times of the year. It is a practice that has been followed for centuries, as our ancestors relied on the availability of seasonal produce to sustain themselves. In recent years, there has been a resurgence of interest in seasonal eating, as people recognize the numerous benefits it offers for both our health and the environment.

When we choose to eat seasonally, we are not only supporting local farmers and businesses, but we are also ensuring that we consume the freshest and most nutrient-rich foods available. Seasonal produce is typically harvested at its peak ripeness, which means it is bursting with flavor and packed with essential vitamins, minerals, and antioxidants. These nutrients are vital for maintaining optimal health and well-being.

One of the key advantages of seasonal eating is the variety it brings to our diet. Each season offers a unique selection of fruits, vegetables, and other foods that are perfectly suited to the climate and conditions of that time of year. For example, in the spring, we can enjoy vibrant greens like asparagus, spinach, and peas, which are rich in vitamins A, C, and K. In the summer, we have an abundance of juicy berries, tomatoes, and melons, which are high in antioxidants and hydrating properties. In the fall, we can savor the earthy flavors of root vegetables like carrots, sweet potatoes, and beets, which are packed with fiber and essential minerals. And in the winter, we can indulge in hearty cruciferous vegetables like broccoli, cauliflower, and Brussels sprouts, which provide us with immune-boosting nutrients.

By embracing seasonal eating, we can also reconnect with nature and the natural rhythms of the earth. Our bodies are designed to adapt to the changing seasons, and by consuming foods that are in sync with the environment, we can enhance our overall well-being. For example, during the colder months, our bodies naturally crave warming and grounding foods like soups, stews, and roasted vegetables. These foods provide us with the nourishment and energy we need to stay healthy and resilient during the winter season.

In addition to the health benefits, seasonal eating also has a positive impact on the environment. When we choose to consume foods that are in season, we reduce the need for long-distance transportation and excessive packaging. This helps to minimize our carbon footprint and support sustainable farming practices. Furthermore, seasonal produce is often grown using fewer pesticides and chemicals, as the crops are naturally more resistant to pests and diseases during their peak growing season. Incorporating seasonal eating into our daily lives can be both enjoyable and practical. Here are some tips to help you get started:

.

Visit your local farmers' market: Farmers' markets are a great place to find a wide variety of seasonal produce. Not only will you be supporting local farmers, but you will also have the opportunity to connect with the people who grow your food and learn more about the different varieties available.

.

.

Join a community-supported agriculture (CSA) program: CSA programs allow you to receive a weekly or monthly box of fresh, locally grown produce directly from a farm. This not only ensures that you have access to seasonal foods, but it also provides you with the opportunity to try new and unique ingredients.

.

.

Plan your meals around seasonal ingredients: Take advantage of the abundance of seasonal produce by incorporating it into your meal planning. Look for recipes that highlight the flavors of the season and experiment with different cooking methods to bring out the best in each ingredient.

.

.

Preserve the harvest: If you come across an abundance of a particular seasonal ingredient, consider preserving it for later use. You can freeze fruits and vegetables, make jams and preserves, or even pickle certain vegetables to enjoy them throughout the year.

.

.

Embrace the flavors of each season: Seasonal eating is not just about the nutritional benefits; it's also about savoring the unique flavors and textures that each season brings. Take the time to appreciate the taste of a perfectly ripe tomato in the summer or the comforting warmth of a bowl of butternut squash soup in the fall.

.

In conclusion, seasonal eating is a simple yet powerful way to enhance our health, support local agriculture, and reduce our impact on the environment. By embracing the natural rhythms of the seasons and incorporating seasonal produce into our diet, we can enjoy a wide variety of nutrient-rich foods while reconnecting with nature and the world around us. So, let's celebrate the flavors and abundance of each season and embark on a journey of seasonal eating for a healthier and more sustainable future.

WHOLE GRAINS

Understanding the Benefits of Whole Grains

Whole grains are an essential component of a nutrient-rich diet. They provide a wide range of health benefits and are packed with essential nutrients that promote overall well-being. Unlike refined grains, which have been stripped of their bran and germ, whole grains retain all parts of the grain, making them a rich source of fiber, vitamins, minerals, and antioxidants.

One of the primary benefits of whole grains is their high fiber content. Fiber plays a crucial role in maintaining a healthy digestive system and preventing constipation. It adds bulk to the stool, making it easier to pass through the intestines. Additionally, fiber helps regulate blood sugar levels, reducing the risk of developing type 2 diabetes. It also aids in weight management by promoting feelings of fullness and preventing overeating.

Whole grains are also rich in vitamins and minerals that are essential for optimal health. For example, whole wheat is a good source of B vitamins, including thiamin, riboflavin, niacin, and folate. These vitamins are involved in energy production, nerve function, and the formation of red blood cells. Other whole grains, such as quinoa and brown rice, provide minerals like magnesium, zinc, and iron, which are necessary for various bodily functions, including bone health, immune system function, and oxygen transport.

In addition to fiber, vitamins, and minerals, whole grains are packed with antioxidants. These powerful compounds help protect the body against oxidative stress and inflammation, which are linked to chronic diseases such as heart disease, cancer, and diabetes. Antioxidants also play a role in maintaining healthy skin and reducing the signs of aging.

Including whole grains in your diet can have a positive impact on heart health. Studies have shown that consuming whole grains regularly can lower the risk of heart disease by reducing cholesterol levels, blood pressure, and inflammation. The fiber and antioxidants in whole grains work together to promote cardiovascular health and protect against the development of heart-related conditions.

Whole grains are also beneficial for weight management. Due to their high fiber content, they provide a feeling of fullness and help control appetite. This can prevent overeating and contribute to maintaining a healthy weight. Additionally, the complex carbohydrates found in whole grains are digested more slowly than refined grains, resulting in a slower release of glucose into the bloodstream. This helps stabilize blood sugar levels and prevents spikes and crashes in energy.

Incorporating whole grains into your meals is easier than you might think. Start by replacing refined grains with whole grain alternatives. For example, choose whole wheat bread instead of white bread, whole grain pasta instead of regular pasta, and brown rice instead of white rice. Experiment with different types of whole grains, such as quinoa, barley, and bulgur, to add variety to your meals.

Here are a few examples of how you can incorporate whole grains into your daily meals:

- Start your day with a bowl of oatmeal topped with fresh berries and a sprinkle of nuts for added crunch and protein.
- Swap out white rice for quinoa or brown rice in your stir-fries or grain bowls.
- Use whole wheat flour instead of refined flour in your baking recipes to make healthier bread, muffins, and pancakes.
- Enjoy a hearty salad with a base of mixed greens and quinoa, topped with roasted vegetables and a drizzle of olive oil and lemon juice.
- Make a nourishing bowl of vegetable soup with barley or farro for added texture and nutrition.

By understanding the benefits of whole grains and incorporating them into your meals, you can enhance the nutrient density of your diet and reap the numerous health benefits they offer. Whole grains are a versatile and delicious addition to any meal, providing a satisfying and nourishing foundation for a nutrient-rich lifestyle.

Different Types of Whole Grains and Their Nutritional Value

Whole grains are an essential component of a nutrient-rich diet. They are packed with essential nutrients, including fiber, vitamins, minerals, and antioxidants, that promote optimal health and well-being. In this section, we will explore the different types of whole grains and their nutritional value, helping you make informed choices when incorporating them into your meals.

Brown Rice: Brown rice is a popular whole grain that is rich in fiber, vitamins, and minerals. Unlike white rice, which has had the bran and germ removed, brown rice retains these nutritious components. It is an excellent source of manganese, selenium, and magnesium, which are essential for maintaining healthy bones, regulating blood sugar levels, and supporting the immune system.

Quinoa: Quinoa is a versatile whole grain that is gluten-free and packed with nutrients. It is a complete protein, meaning it contains all nine essential amino acids necessary for optimal health. Quinoa is also a good source of fiber, iron, magnesium, and phosphorus. It can be used as a base for salads, added to soups, or enjoyed as a side dish.

Oats: Oats are a popular whole grain that is commonly consumed as oatmeal or added to baked goods. They are an excellent source of soluble fiber, which helps lower cholesterol levels and promotes healthy digestion. Oats also contain antioxidants called avenanthramides, which have anti-inflammatory properties and may help reduce the risk of heart disease.

Barley: Barley is a nutritious whole grain that is often used in soups, stews, and salads. It is rich in fiber, vitamins, and minerals, including selenium, copper, and manganese. Barley is also a good source of beta-glucan, a type of soluble fiber that helps lower cholesterol levels and promotes healthy blood sugar control.

Buckwheat: Despite its name, buckwheat is not related to wheat and is naturally gluten-free. It is a nutrient-dense whole grain that is rich in fiber, protein, and essential minerals such as magnesium, copper, and manganese. Buckwheat is commonly used to make flour for pancakes, noodles, and bread.

.

.

Millet: Millet is a gluten-free whole grain that is widely consumed in many parts of the world. It is a good source of fiber, B vitamins, magnesium, and phosphorus. Millet can be cooked and enjoyed as a side dish, added to salads, or used as a base for porridge.

.

.

Whole Wheat: Whole wheat is a staple whole grain that is commonly used to make bread, pasta, and other baked goods. It contains all three parts of the grain: the bran, germ, and endosperm, making it a rich source of fiber, vitamins, and minerals. Whole wheat is also a good source of antioxidants, such as phenolic acids and lignans, which have been linked to a reduced risk of chronic diseases.

.

.

Amaranth: Amaranth is a gluten-free whole grain that is rich in protein, fiber, and essential minerals like calcium, iron, and magnesium. It is also a good source of antioxidants, including vitamin E and phenolic compounds. Amaranth can be cooked and enjoyed as a side dish, added to soups, or used as a thickening agent in recipes.

.

.

Triticale: Triticale is a hybrid grain that is a cross between wheat and rye. It combines the nutritional benefits of both grains, making it a good source of fiber, protein, and essential minerals. Triticale can be used in a variety of recipes, including bread, pasta, and cereals.

.

.

Spelt: Spelt is an ancient whole grain that is closely related to wheat. It is rich in fiber, protein, and essential minerals like manganese and phosphorus. Spelt has a slightly nutty flavor and can be used in a variety of recipes, including bread, pasta, and baked goods.

.

Incorporating a variety of whole grains into your diet can provide a wide range of nutrients and health benefits. Experiment with different types of whole grains in your meals to add variety and maximize your nutrient intake. Whether you enjoy them as a side dish, in salads, or as a base for your favorite recipes, whole grains are a delicious and nutritious addition to any meal.

Incorporating Whole Grains into Your Meals

Whole grains are an essential component of a nutrient-rich diet. They are packed with fiber, vitamins, minerals, and antioxidants that provide numerous health benefits. Incorporating whole grains into your meals not only adds variety and flavor but also boosts the nutritional value of your diet. In this section, we will explore different ways to incorporate whole grains into your meals and provide you with some delicious recipe ideas.

The Versatility of Whole Grains

One of the great things about whole grains is their versatility. They can be used in a wide range of dishes, from breakfast to dinner and even in snacks and desserts. Here are some creative ways to incorporate whole grains into your meals:

.

Breakfast: Start your day with a nutritious and filling breakfast by adding whole grains to your morning routine. Swap out refined grains like white bread or sugary cereals with whole grain options such as oatmeal, whole grain toast, or whole grain cereal. You can also try adding cooked quinoa or amaranth to your smoothies or yogurt bowls for an extra boost of nutrients.

·

·

Lunch: Whole grains can be a great addition to your lunchtime meals. Instead of using white rice or pasta, opt for whole grain alternatives like brown rice, quinoa, or whole wheat pasta. These options provide more fiber and nutrients, keeping you fuller for longer. You can also use whole grain bread or wraps for sandwiches or wraps, adding a delicious and nutritious twist to your midday meal.

·

·

Dinner: Whole grains can be the star of your dinner plate. Experiment with different whole grain options like bulgur, barley, or farro to create hearty and satisfying grain bowls or pilafs. You can also use whole grain breadcrumbs or crushed whole grain cereal as a coating for baked chicken or fish. Another idea is to stuff vegetables like bell peppers or zucchini with a mixture of cooked whole grains, vegetables, and herbs for a flavorful and nutritious dinner option.

·

·

Snacks: Whole grains can also be incorporated into your snacks to keep you energized throughout the day. Instead of reaching for processed snacks, choose whole grain options like air-popped popcorn, whole grain crackers, or homemade granola bars made with whole grain oats. These snacks provide a good source of fiber and nutrients, making them a healthier choice.

·

·

Desserts: Yes, you can even enjoy whole grains in your desserts! Try using whole grain flours like whole wheat flour or oat flour in your baking recipes. You can make whole grain pancakes, muffins, or cookies that are both delicious and nutritious. Adding cooked quinoa or amaranth to your fruit crumbles or puddings can also provide a delightful texture and added nutritional value.

.

Recipe Ideas

Now that you have some ideas on how to incorporate whole grains into your meals, let's explore a few delicious recipe ideas to get you started:

.

Quinoa Salad with Roasted Vegetables: Cook quinoa according to package instructions and let it cool. In a separate pan, roast your favorite vegetables like bell peppers, zucchini, and cherry tomatoes with olive oil, salt, and pepper. Mix the cooked quinoa and roasted vegetables together and add a dressing of your choice, such as lemon vinaigrette or balsamic glaze. This salad can be enjoyed warm or cold and makes a perfect lunch or light dinner option.

.

.

Whole Grain Stir-Fry: Cook brown rice or quinoa and set it aside. In a pan, stir-fry your favorite vegetables like broccoli, carrots, and snap peas with garlic and ginger. Add cooked shrimp, chicken, or tofu for protein. Finally, mix in the cooked whole grains and season with soy sauce or a homemade stir-fry sauce. This quick and easy stir-fry is a nutritious and satisfying dinner option.

.

.

Whole Grain Banana Bread: Mash ripe bananas in a bowl and add whole wheat flour, oats, baking powder, cinnamon, and a touch of honey or maple syrup. Mix until well combined and pour the batter into a greased loaf pan. Bake in a preheated oven at 350°F (175°C) for about 45 minutes or until a toothpick inserted into the center comes out clean. This whole grain banana bread is a healthier alternative to traditional recipes and makes a delicious breakfast or snack.

Remember, the key to incorporating whole grains into your meals is to experiment and have fun with different recipes. By doing so, you can enjoy the nutritional benefits of whole grains while adding variety and flavor to your diet.

Delicious Whole Grain Recipes for Every Meal

Whole grains are an essential part of a nutrient-rich diet. They are packed with fiber, vitamins, minerals, and antioxidants that promote good health and provide sustained energy throughout the day. Incorporating whole grains into your meals not only adds a delicious nutty flavor but also boosts the nutritional value of your dishes. In this section, we will explore some mouthwatering whole grain recipes that you can enjoy for every meal of the day.

Breakfast

Quinoa Breakfast Bowl: Start your day with a nutritious and filling quinoa breakfast bowl. Cook quinoa in almond milk and top it with fresh berries, sliced almonds, and a drizzle of honey. This protein-packed breakfast will keep you energized and satisfied until lunchtime.

Oatmeal Pancakes: Swap your regular pancakes with these wholesome oatmeal pancakes. Blend rolled oats, banana, almond milk, and a pinch of cinnamon to make the batter. Cook them on a non-stick pan and serve with a dollop of Greek yogurt and a sprinkle of chopped nuts.

Lunch

Mediterranean Farro Salad: Combine cooked farro with diced cucumbers, cherry tomatoes, Kalamata olives, feta cheese, and a handful of fresh herbs like parsley and mint. Drizzle with a lemon-olive oil dressing for a refreshing and satisfying lunch option.

·

·

Barley Vegetable Soup: In a large pot, simmer barley with vegetable broth, diced carrots, celery, onions, and your choice of seasonal vegetables. Season with herbs and spices like thyme and bay leaves. This hearty soup is perfect for a comforting and nutritious lunch.

·

Snacks

·

Whole Grain Crackers: Make your own whole grain crackers by combining whole wheat flour, oats, flaxseeds, and a pinch of salt. Roll out the dough, cut into desired shapes, and bake until crispy. Enjoy them with hummus or your favorite dip for a wholesome snack.

·

·

Popcorn Trail Mix: Air-pop some popcorn and mix it with whole grain cereal, dried fruits like cranberries and apricots, and a handful of nuts. This crunchy and sweet snack is packed with fiber and antioxidants.

·

Dinner

·

Quinoa Stuffed Bell Peppers: Cut the tops off bell peppers and remove the seeds. In a skillet, sauté onions, garlic, and your choice of vegetables. Mix in cooked quinoa, tomato sauce, and spices. Stuff the mixture into the bell peppers and bake until tender. This colorful and flavorful dish is a complete meal on its own.

·

Brown Rice Stir-Fry: Cook brown rice according to package instructions. In a wok or skillet, stir-fry your favorite vegetables like broccoli, bell peppers, and snap peas. Add cooked brown rice, soy sauce, and a dash of sesame oil. Toss everything together for a quick and nutritious dinner option.

Dessert

Whole Wheat Banana Bread: Mash ripe bananas and mix them with whole wheat flour, Greek yogurt, honey, and a hint of cinnamon. Bake the batter in a loaf pan until golden and fragrant. This guilt-free banana bread is a perfect way to satisfy your sweet tooth while incorporating whole grains into your dessert.

Quinoa Chocolate Chip Cookies: Combine cooked quinoa with almond flour, dark chocolate chips, coconut oil, and a touch of maple syrup. Form the dough into cookies and bake until golden brown. These chewy and chocolatey cookies are a healthier alternative to traditional cookies.

These recipes are just a starting point to inspire you to incorporate whole grains into your meals. Feel free to experiment with different grains like brown rice, barley, millet, or amaranth, and customize the recipes to suit your taste preferences. By embracing whole grains, you can enjoy delicious and nutritious meals that support your overall health and well-being.

LEAN PROTEIN SOURCES

The Importance of Protein in a Nutrient Rich Diet

Protein is an essential macronutrient that plays a crucial role in our overall health and well-being. It is often referred to as the building block of life, as it is responsible for the growth, repair, and maintenance of tissues in our body. In a nutrient-rich diet, protein holds a special place due to its numerous benefits and its ability to support optimal health.

Protein is made up of amino acids, which are the building blocks that our body uses to create and repair tissues. There are 20 different amino acids, and our body can produce some of them on its own. However, there are nine essential amino acids that our body cannot produce, and we must obtain them through our diet. These essential amino acids are crucial for the proper functioning of our body and are found in various protein-rich foods.

One of the key benefits of protein in a nutrient-rich diet is its role in muscle growth and repair. When we engage in physical activities such as exercise or strength training, our muscles undergo stress and micro-tears. Protein helps in repairing these tears and building new muscle tissue, leading to muscle growth and improved strength. Including an adequate amount of protein in your diet can help support your fitness goals and enhance your athletic performance.

Protein also plays a vital role in weight management. It has a high satiety value, meaning it keeps you feeling full and satisfied for longer periods. This can help curb cravings and prevent overeating, ultimately supporting weight loss or weight maintenance efforts. Additionally, protein has a higher thermic effect compared to carbohydrates and fats, which means that our body burns more calories during the digestion and absorption of protein-rich foods. This can contribute to an increased metabolic rate and improved calorie expenditure.

In addition to its role in muscle growth and weight management, protein is essential for the proper functioning of our immune system. It helps in the production of antibodies, which are proteins that play a crucial role in fighting off infections and diseases. Including adequate protein in your diet can help strengthen your immune system and support overall immune function.

Protein is also involved in the production of enzymes, hormones, and neurotransmitters. Enzymes are proteins that facilitate chemical reactions in our body, while hormones act as messengers that regulate various bodily functions. Neurotransmitters are chemicals that transmit signals between nerve cells, allowing for proper communication within our nervous system. Without sufficient protein intake, these essential processes may be compromised, leading to imbalances and potential health issues.

When it comes to protein sources, there are various options available for both animal-based and plant-based diets. Lean animal protein sources include poultry, fish, lean cuts of beef or pork, and low-fat dairy products. These sources provide high-quality protein along with essential nutrients such as vitamins and minerals. Plant-based protein sources include legumes, tofu, tempeh, quinoa, nuts, and seeds. These sources not only provide protein but also offer additional benefits such as fiber, antioxidants, and healthy fats.

It is important to note that the protein requirements may vary depending on factors such as age, sex, activity level, and overall health. The Recommended Dietary Allowance (RDA) for protein is 0.8 grams per kilogram of body weight for adults. However, athletes, pregnant or lactating women, and individuals recovering from injuries or illnesses may have higher protein needs. Consulting with a healthcare professional or a registered dietitian can help determine the appropriate protein intake for your specific needs.

Incorporating protein-rich foods into your meals can be done in various ways. For example, you can start your day with a protein-packed breakfast by including eggs, Greek yogurt, or a protein smoothie. For lunch and dinner, opt for lean sources of protein such as grilled chicken breast, salmon, or tofu. Snacks can also be protein-focused by choosing options like nuts, seeds, or protein bars. By including protein in each meal and snack, you can ensure that you are meeting your daily protein requirements and reaping the benefits of a nutrient-rich diet.

In conclusion, protein is a vital component of a nutrient-rich diet. It supports muscle growth and repair, aids in weight management, strengthens the immune system, and plays a role in essential bodily functions. Whether you follow an animal-based or plant-based diet, there are numerous protein-rich options available to meet your needs. By incorporating protein into your meals and snacks, you can optimize your health and well-being while enjoying a variety of delicious and nutritious foods.

Lean Animal Protein Sources

Lean animal protein sources are an essential component of a nutrient-rich diet. They provide high-quality protein, along with important vitamins and minerals that support overall health and well-being. Incorporating lean animal protein sources into your meals can help you meet your daily protein needs and promote muscle growth, repair, and maintenance.

When it comes to lean animal protein sources, it's important to choose options that are low in saturated fat and cholesterol. Here are some examples of lean animal protein sources that you can include in your diet:

1. Skinless Chicken Breast

Skinless chicken breast is a popular choice for lean protein. It is low in fat and calories, yet high in protein. Chicken breast is versatile and can be prepared in various ways, such as grilling, baking, or sautéing. It can be used in salads, stir-fries, or as the main protein in a meal.

2. Turkey Breast

Turkey breast is another lean animal protein source that is low in fat and high in protein. It can be used as a substitute for chicken in many recipes. Turkey breast can be roasted, grilled, or used in sandwiches and wraps. It is also a great option for those looking to reduce their red meat consumption.

3. Fish

Fish, such as salmon, tuna, and trout, are excellent sources of lean protein and heart-healthy omega-3 fatty acids. These fatty acids have been shown to have numerous health benefits, including reducing inflammation and improving heart health. Fish can be baked, grilled, or pan-seared and can be enjoyed as a main dish or added to salads and pasta dishes.

4. Lean Beef

While beef is often associated with higher fat content, there are lean cuts available that can be included in a nutrient-rich diet.

Examples of lean beef cuts include sirloin, tenderloin, and eye of round. These cuts are lower in fat and can be prepared by grilling, broiling, or roasting. It's important to trim any visible fat before cooking to reduce the overall fat content.

5. Pork Tenderloin

Pork tenderloin is a lean cut of pork that is low in fat and high in protein. It can be marinated and grilled, roasted, or sautéed. Pork tenderloin is a versatile protein source that can be used in a variety of dishes, from stir-fries to sandwiches.

6. Eggs

Eggs are a complete protein source and can be a part of a nutrient-rich diet. They are versatile and can be prepared in many ways, such as boiled, scrambled, or poached. Eggs can be enjoyed as a standalone meal or added to salads, sandwiches, or stir-fries.

7. Greek Yogurt

Greek yogurt is a protein-rich dairy product that can be included in a nutrient-rich diet. It is lower in sugar and higher in protein compared to regular yogurt. Greek yogurt can be enjoyed on its own, added to smoothies, or used as a substitute for sour cream in recipes.

8. Cottage Cheese

Cottage cheese is another protein-rich dairy product that can be incorporated into a nutrient-rich diet. It is low in fat and carbohydrates and can be enjoyed as a snack or added to salads, smoothies, or baked goods.

9. Low-Fat Milk

Low-fat milk is a good source of protein, calcium, and other essential nutrients. It can be enjoyed on its own or used in recipes such as smoothies, oatmeal, or soups.

10. Lean Deli Meats

When choosing deli meats, opt for lean options such as turkey or chicken breast. These can be used in sandwiches, wraps, or salads for a quick and convenient source of lean protein.

Remember, when incorporating lean animal protein sources

into your diet, it's important to practice portion control and balance your meals with other nutrient-rich foods such as fruits, vegetables, whole grains, and healthy fats. By doing so, you can create a well-rounded and balanced diet that supports your overall health and well-being.

Plant-Based Protein Sources

Plant-based protein sources are an excellent option for individuals looking to incorporate more nutrient-rich foods into their diet. Whether you follow a vegetarian or vegan lifestyle, or simply want to reduce your consumption of animal products, plant-based proteins offer a wide range of health benefits. They are not only rich in essential nutrients but also contribute to a more sustainable and environmentally friendly food system.

The Benefits of Plant-Based Proteins

Plant-based proteins provide numerous health benefits. They are typically lower in saturated fat and cholesterol compared to animal-based proteins, making them heart-healthy choices. Additionally, plant-based proteins are often high in fiber, which aids in digestion and helps maintain a healthy weight. They also contain a variety of vitamins, minerals, and antioxidants that support overall well-being.

Examples of Plant-Based Protein Sources

•

Legumes: Legumes, such as lentils, chickpeas, black beans, and kidney beans, are excellent sources of plant-based protein. They are also rich in fiber, iron, and folate. Legumes can be used in a variety of dishes, including soups, stews, salads, and veggie burgers.

•

•

Quinoa: Quinoa is a complete protein, meaning it contains all nine essential amino acids that the body needs. It is also a good source of fiber, magnesium, and iron. Quinoa can be used as a base for salads, stir-fries, or as a substitute for rice or pasta.

-

-

Tofu and Tempeh: Tofu and tempeh are soy-based products that are popular among vegetarians and vegans. They are versatile and can be used in a variety of dishes, such as stir-fries, curries, and sandwiches. Tofu and tempeh are excellent sources of protein, calcium, and iron.

-

-

Nuts and Seeds: Nuts and seeds, including almonds, walnuts, chia seeds, and hemp seeds, are not only rich in healthy fats but also provide a good amount of protein. They can be enjoyed as a snack, added to smoothies, or used as toppings for salads and yogurt.

-

-

Seitan: Seitan, also known as wheat meat or wheat gluten, is a popular meat substitute among vegetarians and vegans. It is made from gluten, the protein found in wheat. Seitan is high in protein and can be used in a variety of dishes, such as stir-fries, sandwiches, and stews.

-

-

Edamame: Edamame, young soybeans, are a great source of plant-based protein. They are also rich in fiber, folate, and vitamin K. Edamame can be enjoyed as a snack, added to salads, or used in stir-fries.

-

-

Lentils: Lentils are a versatile legume that comes in various colors, including green, red, and black. They are an excellent source of protein, fiber, and folate. Lentils can be used in soups, stews, salads, and even as a meat substitute in dishes like lentil loaf or lentil burgers.

-

-

Chickpeas: Chickpeas, also known as garbanzo beans, are a staple in many cuisines around the world. They are packed with protein, fiber, and essential minerals like iron and magnesium. Chickpeas can be used in salads, hummus, curries, and roasted as a crunchy snack.

.

Incorporating Plant-Based Proteins into Your Meals

Incorporating plant-based proteins into your meals can be both delicious and nutritious. Here are some ideas to help you get started:

- Add legumes, such as black beans or lentils, to your favorite soups or stews for an extra protein boost.
- Use tofu or tempeh in stir-fries, curries, or sandwiches for a meaty texture and protein-packed meal.
- Sprinkle nuts and seeds, like almonds or chia seeds, on top of salads, yogurt, or oatmeal for added crunch and protein.
- Experiment with different grains, such as quinoa or amaranth, as a base for salads or as a side dish.
- Roast chickpeas with your favorite spices for a crunchy and protein-rich snack.
- Incorporate edamame into stir-fries, salads, or enjoy them as a snack on their own.

By incorporating a variety of plant-based protein sources into your meals, you can ensure that you are meeting your nutritional needs while enjoying a diverse and flavorful diet.

Remember, it's important to consult with a healthcare professional or registered dietitian before making any significant changes to your diet, especially if you have specific dietary requirements or health concerns.

Protein-Packed Recipes for a Balanced Diet

Protein is an essential nutrient that plays a crucial role in our overall health and well-being. It is responsible for building and repairing tissues, producing enzymes and hormones, and supporting a healthy immune system. Incorporating protein-rich foods into our diet is essential for maintaining a balanced and nutrient-rich lifestyle. In this section, we will explore some delicious and protein-packed recipes that will not only satisfy your taste buds but also provide you with the necessary nutrients for optimal health.

1. Quinoa and Black Bean Salad

Ingredients:

- 1 cup cooked quinoa
- 1 cup black beans, rinsed and drained
- 1 red bell pepper, diced
- 1 cucumber, diced
- 1/4 cup red onion, finely chopped
- 1/4 cup fresh cilantro, chopped
- Juice of 1 lime
- 2 tablespoons olive oil
- Salt and pepper to taste

Instructions:

- In a large bowl, combine cooked quinoa, black beans, red bell pepper, cucumber, red onion, and cilantro.
- In a small bowl, whisk together lime juice, olive oil, salt, and pepper.
- Pour the dressing over the quinoa mixture and toss until well combined.
- Serve chilled and enjoy as a refreshing and protein-packed salad.

2. Grilled Chicken with Roasted Vegetables

Ingredients:

- 2 boneless, skinless chicken breasts
- 2 tablespoons olive oil
- 1 teaspoon garlic powder
- 1 teaspoon paprika
- Salt and pepper to taste
- 1 zucchini, sliced

- 1 red bell pepper, sliced
- 1 yellow bell pepper, sliced
- 1 red onion, sliced
- 2 tablespoons balsamic vinegar
- Fresh basil leaves for garnish

Instructions:

. Preheat the grill to medium-high heat.

. In a small bowl, mix together olive oil, garlic powder, paprika, salt, and pepper.

. Brush the chicken breasts with the olive oil mixture and place them on the grill. Cook for about 6-8 minutes per side or until the internal temperature reaches 165°F.

. In a separate bowl, toss the sliced zucchini, red bell pepper, yellow bell pepper, and red onion with balsamic vinegar, salt, and pepper.

. Transfer the vegetables to a baking sheet and roast in the oven at 400°F for about 15-20 minutes or until they are tender and slightly caramelized.

. Serve the grilled chicken with the roasted vegetables and garnish with fresh basil leaves for added flavor.

3. Lentil and Vegetable Curry

Ingredients:

- 1 cup dried lentils, rinsed and drained
- 1 tablespoon olive oil
- 1 onion, diced
- 2 cloves garlic, minced
- 1 tablespoon curry powder
- 1 teaspoon ground cumin
- 1 teaspoon ground coriander
- 1/2 teaspoon turmeric
- 1 can (14 oz) diced tomatoes
- 1 can (14 oz) coconut milk
- 2 cups mixed vegetables (such as carrots, peas, and bell peppers)
- Salt and pepper to taste

- Fresh cilantro for garnish

Instructions:

- In a large pot, heat olive oil over medium heat. Add diced onion and minced garlic and sauté until they are soft and fragrant.
- Add curry powder, cumin, coriander, and turmeric to the pot and stir for about a minute to release the flavors.
- Add lentils, diced tomatoes, coconut milk, and mixed vegetables to the pot. Stir well to combine.
- Bring the mixture to a boil, then reduce the heat to low and simmer for about 20-25 minutes or until the lentils are tender.
- Season with salt and pepper to taste.
- Serve the lentil and vegetable curry over cooked rice or with naan bread. Garnish with fresh cilantro for added freshness.

4. Greek Yogurt Parfait

Ingredients:

- 1 cup Greek yogurt
- 1/2 cup granola
- 1/2 cup mixed berries (such as strawberries, blueberries, and raspberries)
- 1 tablespoon honey

Instructions:

- In a glass or a bowl, layer Greek yogurt, granola, and mixed berries.
- Drizzle honey over the top for added sweetness.
- Repeat the layers until all the ingredients are used.
- Serve the Greek yogurt parfait as a protein-packed and nutritious breakfast or snack option.

These protein-packed recipes are just a few examples of how you can incorporate nutrient-rich foods into your diet. By choosing recipes that are high in protein, you can ensure that you are getting the necessary nutrients to support your overall health and well-being. Experiment with different ingredients and flavors to create your own protein-packed meals that are both delicious and nutritious. Remember, a balanced diet is key to maintaining a healthy lifestyle.

HEALTHY FATS, DAIRY AND DAIRY ALTERNATIVES, NUTS AND SEEDS

Understanding the Role of Healthy Fats in Your Diet

Healthy fats play a crucial role in maintaining overall health and well-being. Contrary to popular belief, not all fats are bad for you. In fact, incorporating the right types of fats into your diet can have numerous benefits for your body and mind. This section will explore the importance of healthy fats, their role in your diet, and provide examples of foods that are rich in these beneficial fats.

The Importance of Healthy Fats

Fats are an essential macronutrient that your body needs for various functions. They provide energy, support cell growth, protect organs, and help absorb certain vitamins. Healthy fats, specifically monounsaturated and polyunsaturated fats, have been linked to numerous health benefits, including:

-

Heart Health: Consuming healthy fats can help reduce the risk of heart disease by lowering bad cholesterol levels (LDL) and increasing good cholesterol levels (HDL). This, in turn, can improve overall cardiovascular health.

.

.

Brain Function: Your brain is made up of nearly 60% fat, and it relies on healthy fats to function optimally. Consuming omega-3 fatty acids, found in fatty fish and walnuts, has been associated with improved cognitive function and a reduced risk of age-related cognitive decline.

.

.

Nutrient Absorption: Certain vitamins, such as vitamins A, D, E, and K, are fat-soluble, meaning they require fat to be properly absorbed and utilized by the body. Including healthy fats in your meals can enhance the absorption of these essential vitamins.

.

.

Hormone Regulation: Fats are involved in the production and regulation of hormones in the body. Adequate intake of healthy fats can help maintain hormonal balance, which is crucial for various bodily functions, including metabolism, reproduction, and mood regulation.

.

Examples of Healthy Fats

Now that we understand the importance of healthy fats, let's explore some examples of foods that are rich in these beneficial fats:

.

Avocados: Avocados are a fantastic source of monounsaturated fats, which can help lower bad cholesterol levels. They are also packed with fiber, vitamins, and minerals. Add sliced avocado to salads, spread it on toast, or use it as a creamy base for smoothies.

·

·

Olive Oil: Olive oil is a staple in Mediterranean cuisine and is rich in monounsaturated fats. It has been associated with numerous health benefits, including reducing inflammation and improving heart health. Use olive oil as a dressing for salads or as a cooking oil for sautéing vegetables.

·

·

Fatty Fish: Fatty fish, such as salmon, mackerel, and sardines, are excellent sources of omega-3 fatty acids. These essential fats have been shown to reduce inflammation, support brain health, and promote heart health. Aim to include fatty fish in your diet at least twice a week.

·

·

Nuts and Seeds: Almonds, walnuts, chia seeds, and flaxseeds are all rich in healthy fats, particularly omega-3 fatty acids. They make for convenient and nutritious snacks, or you can sprinkle them on top of salads, yogurt, or oatmeal for an added crunch and nutritional boost.

·

·

Coconut Oil: While coconut oil is high in saturated fat, it contains medium-chain triglycerides (MCTs), which are metabolized differently by the body compared to other saturated fats. MCTs have been associated with increased energy expenditure and may aid in weight management. Use coconut oil sparingly in cooking or baking.

·

·

Nut Butter: Natural nut butters, such as almond butter or peanut butter, are excellent sources of healthy fats. They can be spread on whole grain toast, added to smoothies, or used as a dip for fruits and vegetables.

·

. Seeds: Sunflower seeds, pumpkin seeds, and sesame seeds are all rich in healthy fats, fiber, and various minerals. Sprinkle them on salads, yogurt, or incorporate them into homemade granola or energy bars.

. Remember, while healthy fats offer numerous benefits, moderation is key. Fats are calorie-dense, so it's important to consume them in appropriate portions as part of a balanced diet. Aim to replace unhealthy fats, such as saturated and trans fats found in processed foods and fried items, with healthier alternatives.

By incorporating these examples of healthy fats into your diet, you can reap the benefits of improved heart health, enhanced brain function, and overall well-being. Experiment with different recipes and meal ideas to make your meals both nutritious and delicious.

Choosing Healthy Dairy and Dairy Alternatives

When it comes to incorporating nutrient-rich foods into your diet, dairy and dairy alternatives play a significant role. These food options provide essential nutrients like calcium, protein, and vitamins, which are crucial for maintaining optimal health. In this section, we will explore the various options available and provide guidance on choosing healthy dairy and dairy alternatives.

Understanding the Importance of Dairy and Dairy Alternatives

Dairy products are well-known for their high calcium content, which is essential for strong bones and teeth. Additionally, dairy is a good source of protein, vitamins (such as vitamin D and vitamin B12), and minerals like phosphorus and potassium. However, some individuals may have lactose intolerance or choose to follow a dairy-free lifestyle due to personal preferences or dietary restrictions. In such cases, dairy alternatives become a valuable option.

Exploring Dairy Alternatives

Dairy alternatives are plant-based products that mimic the taste and texture of dairy products. They are typically made from nuts, seeds, legumes, or grains and offer a range of nutritional benefits. Some popular dairy alternatives include:

•

Almond Milk: Made from ground almonds and water, almond milk is a popular dairy alternative. It is low in calories and contains no cholesterol. Almond milk is often fortified with calcium and vitamin D to match the nutritional profile of dairy milk.

•

•

Soy Milk: Soy milk is made from soybeans and is a great source of protein. It is also rich in calcium, vitamin D, and other essential nutrients. Soy milk is a versatile option and can be used in various recipes and beverages.

•

•

Coconut Milk: Coconut milk is derived from the flesh of mature coconuts. It has a creamy texture and a slightly sweet taste. While coconut milk is higher in calories compared to other dairy alternatives, it is a good source of healthy fats and provides important nutrients like iron and magnesium.

•

•

Oat Milk: Oat milk is made from soaked oats blended with water. It has a mild, slightly sweet flavor and a creamy consistency. Oat milk is often fortified with vitamins and minerals, making it a nutritious choice.

•

•

Rice Milk: Rice milk is made from milled rice and water. It has a naturally sweet taste and is often fortified with calcium and vitamin D. Rice milk is a suitable option for individuals with allergies or intolerances to nuts, soy, or gluten.

.

.

Hemp Milk: Hemp milk is made from hemp seeds and water. It is a rich source of omega-3 fatty acids, protein, and essential minerals. Hemp milk has a slightly nutty flavor and can be a great addition to smoothies or cereal.

.

Choosing Healthy Dairy Products

If you consume dairy products, it is important to choose wisely to ensure you are getting the most nutritional benefits. Here are some tips for selecting healthy dairy options:

.

Opt for Low-Fat or Skim Varieties: Choose low-fat or skim milk, yogurt, and cheese to reduce your intake of saturated fats. These options still provide the same essential nutrients but with fewer calories and less fat.

.

.

Look for Fortified Products: Some dairy products, such as milk and yogurt, are fortified with additional nutrients like vitamin D and calcium. Check the labels to ensure you are choosing products that offer these added benefits.

.

.

Choose Plain and Unsweetened: Flavored dairy products often contain added sugars, which can contribute to excess calorie intake. Opt for plain and unsweetened varieties and add your own natural sweeteners or fruits for flavor.

.

.

Consider Organic Options: Organic dairy products come from animals raised without the use of antibiotics or hormones. Choosing organic options can help reduce your exposure to potentially harmful substances.

.

.

Read Labels: Pay attention to the ingredient list and nutritional information on dairy products. Avoid products that contain excessive additives, preservatives, or artificial sweeteners.

.

Remember, moderation is key when consuming dairy products. While they offer valuable nutrients, excessive intake can contribute to high calorie and saturated fat intake. Aim for a balanced approach and incorporate a variety of nutrient-rich foods into your diet.

By choosing healthy dairy products or dairy alternatives, you can enjoy the benefits of these nutrient-rich options while catering to your personal preferences or dietary needs. Experiment with different alternatives and find the ones that suit your taste and nutritional requirements.

The Nutritional Benefits of Nuts and Seeds

Nuts and seeds are not only delicious and versatile, but they also offer a wide range of nutritional benefits. Packed with essential nutrients, healthy fats, and fiber, nuts and seeds are a valuable addition to any nutrient-rich diet. Whether you enjoy them as a snack, sprinkle them on salads, or incorporate them into your favorite recipes, nuts and seeds can provide numerous health benefits.

Nutrient Profile

Nuts and seeds are nutrient powerhouses, containing a variety of vitamins, minerals, and antioxidants. While the nutrient composition varies slightly between different types of nuts and seeds, they generally share some common nutritional characteristics.

One of the key nutrients found in nuts and seeds is healthy fats. These include monounsaturated and polyunsaturated fats, such as omega-3 and omega-6 fatty acids. These fats are essential for brain health, heart health, and overall well-being. Additionally, nuts and seeds are excellent sources of protein, making them a valuable option for vegetarians and vegans.

Nuts and seeds are also rich in fiber, which plays a crucial role in maintaining a healthy digestive system and promoting feelings of fullness. Fiber can help regulate blood sugar levels, lower cholesterol levels, and support weight management.

Furthermore, nuts and seeds are packed with vitamins and minerals. For example, almonds are a great source of vitamin E, magnesium, and calcium. Walnuts are rich in omega-3 fatty acids and antioxidants. Chia seeds are high in fiber, omega-3 fatty acids, and calcium. Pumpkin seeds are an excellent source of iron, zinc, and magnesium. These are just a few examples of the diverse nutrient profiles found in nuts and seeds.

Heart Health

Incorporating nuts and seeds into your diet can have a positive impact on heart health. The healthy fats found in nuts and seeds, such as monounsaturated and polyunsaturated fats, can help lower LDL (bad) cholesterol levels and reduce the risk of heart disease. Additionally, the high levels of antioxidants found in nuts and seeds can help reduce inflammation and oxidative stress, both of which are linked to heart disease.

Several studies have shown that regular consumption of nuts, such as almonds and walnuts, can lower the risk of heart disease. For example, a study published in the New England Journal of Medicine found that individuals who consumed nuts at least five times a week had a significantly lower risk of heart disease compared to those who rarely ate nuts.

Weight Management

Contrary to popular belief, incorporating nuts and seeds into your diet can actually support weight management. Despite being calorie-dense, the combination of healthy fats, protein, and fiber in nuts and seeds can help promote feelings of fullness and reduce overall calorie intake.

Research has shown that individuals who regularly consume nuts and seeds tend to have a lower body mass index (BMI) and a reduced risk of obesity. A study published in the American Journal of Clinical Nutrition found that individuals who included nuts in their diet had a lower risk of weight gain over a five-year period compared to those who rarely ate nuts.

Blood Sugar Control

Nuts and seeds can also play a role in blood sugar control, making them a valuable addition to the diets of individuals with diabetes or those at risk of developing the condition. The combination of healthy fats, protein, and fiber in nuts and seeds helps slow down the absorption of carbohydrates, preventing rapid spikes in blood sugar levels.

Several studies have demonstrated the beneficial effects of nuts and seeds on blood sugar control. For example, a study published in the Journal of the American College of Nutrition found that individuals with type 2 diabetes who consumed two ounces of nuts daily experienced improved blood sugar control and reduced insulin resistance.

Brain Health

The nutrients found in nuts and seeds can also support brain health and cognitive function. The omega-3 fatty acids, antioxidants, and vitamin E present in nuts and seeds have been linked to a reduced risk of cognitive decline and improved brain function.

A study published in the Journal of Nutrition, Health & Aging found that individuals who consumed nuts and seeds regularly had a lower risk of developing Alzheimer's disease and age-related cognitive decline. The researchers attributed these benefits to the high levels of antioxidants and healthy fats found in nuts and seeds.

Incorporating Nuts and Seeds into Your Diet

There are numerous ways to incorporate nuts and seeds into your daily meals and snacks. Here are some ideas to get you started:

- Add a handful of mixed nuts to your morning cereal or yogurt.
- Sprinkle chia seeds or flaxseeds on top of your salads or smoothies.
- Use almond flour or ground flaxseeds as a substitute for traditional flour in baking recipes.
- Enjoy a handful of trail mix as a convenient and nutritious snack.
- Make your own nut butter by blending your favorite nuts in a food processor.
- Use crushed nuts as a coating for baked chicken or fish.
- Add sesame seeds or sunflower seeds to stir-fries or roasted vegetables.

Remember to choose unsalted and unflavored varieties of nuts and seeds to avoid excessive sodium or added sugars.

In conclusion, nuts and seeds are a valuable addition to a nutrient-rich diet. They offer a wide range of health benefits, including improved heart health, weight management, blood sugar control, and brain health. By incorporating a variety of nuts and seeds into your meals and snacks, you can enjoy their delicious flavors while reaping the nutritional rewards they provide.

Incorporating Healthy Fats, Dairy Alternatives, Nuts, and Seeds into Your Meals

Incorporating healthy fats, dairy alternatives, nuts, and seeds into your meals is a great way to enhance the nutrient density of your diet. These food groups provide essential nutrients, such as omega-3 fatty acids, calcium, and protein, that are important for overall health and well-being. By including a variety of these foods in your meals, you can add flavor, texture, and nutritional value to your dishes.

Healthy Fats

Healthy fats are an essential part of a balanced diet. They provide energy, support cell growth, and help the body absorb certain vitamins. Some examples of healthy fats include avocados, olive oil, nuts, and seeds. Here are a few ways you can incorporate healthy fats into your meals:

-

Avocado: Mash avocado and spread it on whole grain toast for a nutritious and satisfying breakfast. You can also add sliced avocado to salads, sandwiches, or wraps for a creamy texture and added flavor.

-

-

Olive Oil: Use olive oil as a dressing for salads or as a cooking oil for sautéing vegetables. It adds a rich flavor to your dishes and provides heart-healthy monounsaturated fats.

-

-

Nuts and Seeds: Sprinkle a handful of nuts or seeds on top of your yogurt, oatmeal, or smoothie bowl for added crunch and nutritional value. You can also use them as a topping for salads or incorporate them into homemade granola or energy bars.

-

Dairy Alternatives

If you follow a dairy-free or vegan diet, there are plenty of alternatives available that can provide similar nutritional benefits. Here are some examples of dairy alternatives and how you can incorporate them into your meals:

-

Plant-Based Milk: Replace cow's milk with plant-based alternatives such as almond milk, soy milk, or oat milk. These can be used in smoothies, cereal, or baking recipes as a substitute for regular milk.

.

.

Yogurt Alternatives: Opt for dairy-free yogurts made from coconut milk, almond milk, or soy milk. Enjoy them on their own, or use them as a base for smoothie bowls, parfaits, or salad dressings.

.

.

Cheese Alternatives: There are various dairy-free cheese alternatives available, made from ingredients like nuts, soy, or tapioca starch. Use them in recipes that call for cheese, such as pizzas, sandwiches, or pasta dishes.

.

Nuts and Seeds

Nuts and seeds are packed with essential nutrients, including healthy fats, protein, fiber, vitamins, and minerals. They can be enjoyed as a snack on their own or incorporated into meals in various ways:

.

Trail Mix: Create your own trail mix by combining a variety of nuts and seeds, along with dried fruits and a sprinkle of dark chocolate chips. This portable snack is perfect for on-the-go or as a mid-afternoon pick-me-up.

.

.

Nut Butters: Spread almond butter, peanut butter, or cashew butter on whole grain bread or use them as a dip for apple slices or celery sticks. Nut butters can also be added to smoothies or used as a base for homemade energy balls.

.

.

Seeds: Sprinkle chia seeds, flaxseeds, or hemp seeds on top of your yogurt, oatmeal, or salads for an added nutritional boost. You can also use them in baking recipes, such as muffins or bread.

.

Incorporating Healthy Fats, Dairy Alternatives, Nuts, and Seeds into Your Meals

Now that you have some ideas on how to incorporate healthy fats, dairy alternatives, nuts, and seeds into your meals, it's time to get creative in the kitchen. Here are a few meal ideas that showcase the versatility of these nutrient-rich ingredients:

.

Quinoa Salad with Avocado and Mixed Nuts: Cook quinoa according to package instructions and let it cool. In a bowl, combine cooked quinoa, diced avocado, mixed nuts (such as almonds, walnuts, and pistachios), chopped fresh herbs (such as parsley or cilantro), and a squeeze of lemon juice. Season with salt and pepper to taste. This salad can be enjoyed as a light lunch or a side dish.

.

.

Vegan Stir-Fry with Tofu and Cashews: In a wok or large skillet, heat some olive oil and sauté diced tofu until golden brown. Add your favorite vegetables, such as bell peppers, broccoli, and snap peas, and stir-fry until tender-crisp. In a small bowl, whisk together soy sauce, sesame oil, and a touch of maple syrup. Pour the sauce over the stir-fry and toss to coat. Serve over brown rice or quinoa and sprinkle with cashews for added crunch.

.

.

Chia Pudding with Berries and Almond Butter: In a jar or bowl, mix together chia seeds, plant-based milk (such as almond milk or coconut milk), and a touch of sweetener (such as maple syrup or honey). Stir well and let it sit in the refrigerator overnight to thicken. In the morning, top the chia pudding with fresh berries, a drizzle of almond butter, and a sprinkle of granola for a nutritious and satisfying breakfast.

.

Remember, incorporating healthy fats, dairy alternatives, nuts, and seeds into your meals is all about variety and balance. Experiment with different flavors and textures to find combinations that you enjoy. By doing so, you'll not only enhance the nutritional value of your meals but also add deliciousness to your plate.

NUTRIENT RICH SNACKING

The Importance of Nutrient Rich Snacks

Snacking is a common part of our daily routine, and it can either contribute to our overall health or hinder our progress towards a nutrient-rich diet. When we think of snacks, we often envision unhealthy options like chips, cookies, or candy. However, incorporating nutrient-rich snacks into our diet can have numerous benefits for our health and well-being.

One of the primary reasons why nutrient-rich snacks are important is that they provide us with essential nutrients that our bodies need to function properly. These snacks are typically packed with vitamins, minerals, fiber, and other beneficial compounds that support our overall health. By choosing snacks that are rich in nutrients, we can ensure that our bodies receive the necessary fuel to perform at their best.

Nutrient-rich snacks also help to stabilize our blood sugar levels throughout the day. When we consume snacks that are high in refined sugars or carbohydrates, our blood sugar levels spike, leading to a sudden burst of energy followed by a crash. This rollercoaster effect can leave us feeling tired, irritable, and craving more unhealthy snacks. On the other hand, nutrient-rich snacks provide a steady release of energy, keeping us satisfied and energized for longer periods.

In addition to providing essential nutrients and stabilizing blood sugar levels, nutrient-rich snacks can also aid in weight management. When we choose snacks that are high in nutrients and low in empty calories, we feel more satisfied and less likely to overeat during our main meals. These snacks can help curb cravings, reduce mindless snacking, and contribute to a balanced diet.

Furthermore, nutrient-rich snacks can support our immune system and help prevent illness. Many fruits, vegetables, nuts, and seeds are rich in antioxidants, which play a crucial role in protecting our cells from damage caused by free radicals. By incorporating these snacks into our diet, we can boost our immune system and reduce the risk of chronic diseases.

Now that we understand the importance of nutrient-rich snacks, let's explore some healthy snack ideas that cater to different cravings and dietary preferences:

- **Craving something sweet?** Opt for a bowl of mixed berries, a sliced apple with almond butter, or a homemade fruit smoothie with Greek yogurt.

-

- **Need a savory fix?** Try roasted chickpeas, air-popped popcorn seasoned with herbs and spices, or a handful of mixed nuts and seeds.

-

- **Looking for a protein boost?** Snack on hard-boiled eggs, Greek yogurt with berries, or a small portion of lean deli meat with whole grain crackers.

·

·

Want something crunchy? Enjoy carrot sticks with hummus, cucumber slices with tzatziki, or kale chips baked with olive oil and sea salt.

·

·

Craving a creamy treat? Indulge in a small portion of avocado on whole grain toast, a chia seed pudding made with almond milk, or a homemade smoothie bowl topped with nuts and seeds.

·

Remember, portion control is key when it comes to snacking. While nutrient-rich snacks are beneficial for our health, it's important to enjoy them in moderation. Be mindful of your portion sizes and listen to your body's hunger and fullness cues. Incorporating nutrient-rich snacks into our daily routine doesn't have to be complicated. With a little planning and preparation, we can make healthier choices that support our overall well-being. By choosing nutrient-rich snacks, we can nourish our bodies, satisfy our cravings, and maintain a balanced diet. So, the next time you reach for a snack, think about the nutrients it provides and choose wisely for a healthier you.

Healthy Snack Ideas for Every Craving

When it comes to snacking, it's important to choose options that not only satisfy your cravings but also provide your body with essential nutrients. Nutrient-rich snacks can help keep your energy levels stable, curb hunger between meals, and support overall health. In this section, we will explore a variety of healthy snack ideas for every craving, ensuring that you have plenty of options to choose from.

1. Crunchy Snacks:

- Raw vegetables with hummus or Greek yogurt dip
- Baked kale chips seasoned with sea salt and olive oil
- Roasted chickpeas with spices like paprika or cumin
- Air-popped popcorn sprinkled with nutritional yeast or cinnamon
- Rice cakes topped with almond butter and sliced bananas

2. Sweet Snacks:

- Fresh fruit salad with a drizzle of honey or a sprinkle of cinnamon
- Greek yogurt parfait with layers of berries and granola
- Homemade energy balls made with dates, nuts, and seeds
- Dark chocolate squares paired with a handful of almonds
- Frozen grapes or banana slices dipped in melted dark chocolate

3. Savory Snacks:

- Whole grain crackers topped with avocado and cherry tomatoes
- Mini caprese skewers with cherry tomatoes, mozzarella, and basil
- Sliced cucumbers with smoked salmon and cream cheese
- Edamame beans lightly salted and steamed
- Roasted seaweed sheets for a satisfying umami flavor

4. Protein-Packed Snacks:

- Hard-boiled eggs sprinkled with sea salt and black pepper

- Cottage cheese with sliced peaches or pineapple
- Turkey or chicken roll-ups with lettuce and mustard
- Greek yogurt with a handful of mixed nuts and berries
- Tuna or salmon salad lettuce wraps for a quick and filling snack

5. Energy-Boosting Snacks:

- Trail mix with a combination of nuts, seeds, and dried fruits
- Apple slices spread with almond butter and sprinkled with chia seeds
- Smoothie made with spinach, banana, almond milk, and a scoop of protein powder
- Quinoa salad with diced vegetables and a lemon vinaigrette dressing
- Chia seed pudding topped with fresh berries and a drizzle of honey

6. Comforting Snacks:

- Whole grain toast with mashed avocado and a sprinkle of sea salt
- Warm oatmeal topped with sliced almonds and a dollop of Greek yogurt
- Baked sweet potato fries seasoned with herbs and spices
- Homemade vegetable soup with a side of whole grain crackers
- Grilled cheese sandwich made with whole grain bread and low-fat cheese

7. Hydrating Snacks:

- Watermelon slices for a refreshing and hydrating snack
- Cucumber slices with a squeeze of lemon juice and a sprinkle of chili powder
- Coconut water blended with frozen berries for

a delicious smoothie

- Homemade fruit popsicles made with pureed fruits and coconut water
- Chilled green tea infused with fresh mint leaves and a splash of lime juice

Remember, the key to healthy snacking is to choose options that are nutrient-dense and provide a balance of macronutrients. Incorporating a variety of fruits, vegetables, whole grains, lean proteins, and healthy fats into your snacks will ensure that you are fueling your body with the necessary nutrients it needs to thrive.

By planning ahead and having these healthy snack options readily available, you can avoid reaching for processed and unhealthy choices. Experiment with different combinations and flavors to find the snacks that satisfy your cravings while nourishing your body. With these healthy snack ideas, you can enjoy guilt-free snacking and support your overall health and well-being.

Snack Recipes for Sustained Energy and Nutrition

When it comes to snacking, it's important to choose options that not only satisfy your cravings but also provide sustained energy and essential nutrients. In this section, we will explore some delicious and nutritious snack recipes that will keep you fueled throughout the day.

Energy-Boosting Trail Mix

Trail mix is a classic snack that is not only convenient but also packed with energy-boosting ingredients. You can create your own trail mix by combining a variety of nuts, seeds, dried fruits, and a touch of sweetness. Here's a simple recipe to get you started:

Ingredients:

- 1 cup almonds

- 1 cup cashews
- 1 cup pumpkin seeds
- 1 cup dried cranberries
- 1/2 cup dark chocolate chips
- 1/4 cup honey or maple syrup
- 1 teaspoon cinnamon

Instructions:

- Preheat your oven to 350°F (175°C).
- In a large bowl, combine the almonds, cashews, pumpkin seeds, dried cranberries, and dark chocolate chips.
- Drizzle the honey or maple syrup over the mixture and sprinkle with cinnamon. Stir well to ensure all ingredients are coated.
- Spread the mixture evenly on a baking sheet and bake for 10-15 minutes, or until lightly toasted.
- Allow the trail mix to cool completely before transferring it to an airtight container.
- Enjoy a handful of this energy-boosting trail mix whenever you need a quick pick-me-up.

Protein-Packed Greek Yogurt Parfait

Greek yogurt is an excellent source of protein and makes for a satisfying and nutritious snack. By layering it with fruits and nuts, you can create a delicious and balanced parfait. Here's a simple recipe to try:

Ingredients:

- 1 cup Greek yogurt
- 1/2 cup mixed berries (such as strawberries, blueberries, and raspberries)
- 1/4 cup granola
- 2 tablespoons chopped nuts (such as almonds or walnuts)
- 1 tablespoon honey or maple syrup (optional)

Instructions:

- In a glass or bowl, layer half of the Greek yogurt.
- Add a layer of mixed berries on top of the yogurt.

- Sprinkle half of the granola and chopped nuts over the berries.
- Repeat the layers with the remaining Greek yogurt, berries, granola, and nuts.
- Drizzle with honey or maple syrup, if desired.
- Enjoy this protein-packed Greek yogurt parfait as a mid-morning or afternoon snack.

Veggie Sticks with Hummus

Crunchy and refreshing, veggie sticks paired with hummus make for a nutritious and satisfying snack. You can choose a variety of vegetables such as carrots, celery, bell peppers, and cucumber. Here's a simple recipe for homemade hummus:

Ingredients:

- 1 can chickpeas, drained and rinsed
- 2 tablespoons tahini
- 2 tablespoons lemon juice
- 1 clove garlic, minced
- 2 tablespoons olive oil
- Salt and pepper to taste

Instructions:

- In a food processor, combine the chickpeas, tahini, lemon juice, garlic, olive oil, salt, and pepper.
- Blend until smooth and creamy, adding a little water if needed to achieve the desired consistency.
- Transfer the hummus to a serving bowl.
- Wash and cut your choice of vegetables into sticks.
- Serve the veggie sticks alongside the homemade hummus for a nutritious and satisfying snack.

Quinoa Energy Balls

Quinoa is a nutrient-rich grain that is packed with protein, fiber, and essential minerals. By combining it with other wholesome ingredients, you can create energy balls that are perfect for a quick and nutritious snack. Here's a simple recipe to try:

Ingredients:

- 1 cup cooked quinoa

- 1/2 cup almond butter
- 1/4 cup honey or maple syrup
- 1/4 cup unsweetened shredded coconut
- 1/4 cup dark chocolate chips
- 1 teaspoon vanilla extract
- Pinch of salt

Instructions:

- In a large bowl, combine the cooked quinoa, almond butter, honey or maple syrup, shredded coconut, dark chocolate chips, vanilla extract, and salt.
- Stir well until all ingredients are evenly mixed.
- Using your hands, roll the mixture into small balls, about 1 inch in diameter.
- Place the energy balls on a baking sheet lined with parchment paper.
- Refrigerate for at least 30 minutes to allow the balls to firm up.
- Store the quinoa energy balls in an airtight container in the refrigerator for up to one week.
- Enjoy one or two energy balls whenever you need a quick and nutritious snack.

These snack recipes are just a starting point to inspire you to create your own nutrient-rich snacks. Remember to choose ingredients that are rich in essential nutrients and provide sustained energy to keep you going throughout the day. Happy snacking!

Smart Snacking Tips for a Nutrient Rich Lifestyle

Snacking can often be seen as a guilty pleasure or a mindless habit, but when done right, it can actually contribute to a nutrient-rich lifestyle. Smart snacking involves choosing snacks that are not only delicious but also packed with essential nutrients to fuel your body and keep you satisfied between meals. In this section, we will explore some tips and strategies for smart snacking that will help you maintain a nutrient-rich lifestyle.

1. Plan Ahead

One of the keys to successful snacking is planning ahead. By taking the time to plan your snacks in advance, you can ensure that you have healthy options readily available when hunger strikes. Consider setting aside some time each week to prepare and portion out your snacks. This could involve chopping up fruits and vegetables, portioning out nuts and seeds, or making homemade energy bars. By having these snacks on hand, you'll be less likely to reach for unhealthy options when hunger strikes.

2. Choose Nutrient-Dense Snacks

When it comes to snacking, not all foods are created equal. Instead of reaching for empty-calorie snacks like chips or cookies, opt for nutrient-dense options that provide a good balance of macronutrients (carbohydrates, protein, and fats) as well as essential vitamins and minerals. Some examples of nutrient-dense snacks include:

- Greek yogurt with berries and a sprinkle of nuts
- Hummus with carrot sticks or whole grain crackers
- Apple slices with almond butter
- Hard-boiled eggs
- Trail mix with dried fruits and nuts
- Homemade energy balls made with oats, nut butter, and seeds

These snacks not only provide a satisfying crunch or sweetness but also offer a range of nutrients that will keep you energized and nourished.

3. Incorporate Protein

Protein is an essential macronutrient that plays a crucial role in maintaining and repairing tissues, supporting immune function, and promoting satiety. Including protein-rich snacks in your daily routine can help keep you feeling full and satisfied between meals. Some protein-rich snack ideas include:

- Greek yogurt or cottage cheese with fruit
- Edamame or roasted chickpeas
- Sliced turkey or chicken breast wrapped in lettuce
- Protein smoothie made with a scoop of protein powder, fruits, and vegetables
- Hard-boiled eggs or egg muffins
- Nut butter spread on whole grain toast or apple slices

By incorporating protein into your snacks, you'll not only satisfy your hunger but also support your body's overall health and well-being.

4. Focus on Fiber

Fiber is another important nutrient that plays a key role in maintaining a healthy digestive system, regulating blood sugar levels, and promoting feelings of fullness. Including fiber-rich snacks in your daily routine can help keep you satisfied and prevent overeating. Some fiber-rich snack ideas include:

- Raw vegetables with hummus or guacamole
- Fresh fruits like apples, pears, or berries
- Whole grain crackers or rice cakes with nut butter
- Popcorn (air-popped or lightly seasoned)
- Chia seed pudding or overnight oats
- Roasted chickpeas or lentil chips

These snacks not only provide a good source of fiber but also offer a variety of textures and flavors to keep your taste buds satisfied.

5. Stay Hydrated

Sometimes, what we perceive as hunger is actually thirst. Before reaching for a snack, try drinking a glass of water and wait for a few minutes to see if your hunger subsides. Staying hydrated is essential for overall health and can help prevent unnecessary snacking. If you find plain water boring, try infusing it with fruits or herbs for a refreshing twist.

6. Practice Mindful Snacking

Mindful snacking involves being fully present and aware of your eating habits. Instead of mindlessly munching on snacks while watching TV or working, take the time to savor and enjoy each bite. Pay attention to the flavors, textures, and sensations of the food. This practice can help you tune in to your body's hunger and fullness cues, preventing overeating and promoting a healthier relationship with food.

7. Portion Control

While snacking can be a healthy habit, it's important to practice portion control to avoid consuming excess calories. Even nutrient-rich snacks can contribute to weight gain if consumed in large quantities. Consider portioning out your snacks in advance or using smaller plates or bowls to help control your portion sizes.

8. Listen to Your Body

Lastly, listen to your body's cues and eat when you're truly hungry. Snacking should be a response to physical hunger rather than emotional or boredom-driven cravings. Pay attention to your body's signals of hunger and fullness, and honor them by choosing nutritious snacks that will nourish and satisfy you.

By incorporating these smart snacking tips into your daily routine, you can enjoy the benefits of a nutrient-rich lifestyle. Remember, snacking can be a positive and enjoyable part of your diet when done mindfully and with a focus on nourishing your body.

MEAL PLANNING WITH NUTRIENT RICH FOODS

The Benefits of Meal Planning

Meal planning is a powerful tool that can greatly enhance your journey towards a nutrient-rich lifestyle. By taking the time to plan your meals in advance, you can ensure that you are consistently nourishing your body with the right balance of nutrients. In this section, we will explore the numerous benefits of meal planning and how it can positively impact your overall health and well-being.

1. Saves Time and Effort

One of the primary advantages of meal planning is that it saves you valuable time and effort in the long run. By dedicating a specific time each week to plan your meals, you eliminate the need to constantly think about what to cook or eat. This can be especially beneficial for individuals with busy schedules or those who find themselves frequently resorting to unhealthy convenience foods due to lack of time. With a well-thought-out meal plan, you can streamline your grocery shopping, prep ingredients in advance, and have a clear roadmap for your meals throughout the week.

2. Promotes Healthier Food Choices

When you have a meal plan in place, you are more likely to make healthier food choices. By carefully selecting nutrient-rich ingredients and incorporating a variety of fruits, vegetables, whole grains, lean proteins, and healthy fats into your meals, you can ensure that your body receives the essential nutrients it needs to thrive. Meal planning allows you to be intentional about your food choices and helps you avoid impulsive decisions that may lead to less nutritious options.

For example, if your meal plan includes a balanced mix of colorful vegetables, lean proteins, and whole grains, you are less likely to reach for processed snacks or fast food when hunger strikes. Instead, you can rely on your pre-planned meals and snacks to provide you with sustained energy and optimal nutrition.

3. Supports Weight Management Goals

Meal planning can be a valuable tool for individuals looking to manage their weight. By carefully portioning your meals and snacks and incorporating a balance of macronutrients, you can better control your caloric intake and ensure that you are not overeating. Additionally, meal planning allows you to include a variety of nutrient-dense foods that can help you feel satisfied and prevent unnecessary cravings or mindless snacking.

For instance, if your goal is to lose weight, you can create a meal plan that includes a calorie deficit while still providing all the necessary nutrients. On the other hand, if your goal is to maintain or gain weight, you can adjust your meal plan accordingly to include more calorie-dense foods without compromising on nutrient quality.

4. Reduces Food Waste

Another significant benefit of meal planning is that it helps reduce food waste. When you plan your meals in advance, you can make a comprehensive grocery list based on the ingredients you will need for the week. This ensures that you only purchase what you need and minimizes the chances of buying excess perishable items that may go to waste.

Moreover, meal planning allows you to repurpose ingredients and leftovers creatively. For example, if you plan to make a roasted chicken for dinner, you can incorporate the leftover chicken into a salad or wrap for lunch the next day. This not only reduces food waste but also saves you money in the long run.

5. Enhances Variety and Culinary Exploration

Meal planning provides an opportunity to explore new recipes and experiment with different flavors and cuisines. By incorporating a diverse range of nutrient-rich foods into your meal plan, you can expand your culinary horizons and discover exciting ways to nourish your body.

For instance, you can dedicate one day of the week to trying a new recipe that features a superfood or an antioxidant-rich ingredient. This not only adds variety to your meals but also exposes you to a wider range of nutrients and flavors.

6. Supports Stress Management

In today's fast-paced world, stress can take a toll on our overall well-being. Meal planning can help alleviate some of that stress by providing structure and organization to your meals. When you have a clear plan in place, you can eliminate the last-minute scramble to figure out what to eat, which can be particularly stressful after a long day.

Additionally, meal planning allows you to allocate time for meal preparation in advance. By prepping ingredients or even cooking meals ahead of time, you can reduce the stress associated with cooking during busy weekdays. This can be especially beneficial for individuals who find cooking to be a therapeutic activity but struggle to find time for it on a daily basis.

7. Saves Money

Meal planning can also help you save money on your grocery bills. When you plan your meals in advance, you can make a comprehensive shopping list and avoid impulse purchases. By sticking to your list and buying only what you need, you can minimize food waste and reduce the chances of buying unnecessary items that may go unused.

Furthermore, meal planning allows you to take advantage of sales and discounts. By planning your meals around seasonal produce or items that are on sale, you can maximize your budget and still enjoy a wide variety of nutrient-rich foods.

In conclusion, meal planning offers numerous benefits that can greatly enhance your nutrient-rich lifestyle. From saving time and effort to promoting healthier food choices and supporting weight management goals, meal planning is a powerful tool that can positively impact your overall health and well-being. By incorporating meal planning into your routine, you can ensure that you consistently nourish your body with the right balance of nutrients and set yourself up for success on your journey towards optimal health.

Creating a Nutrient Rich Meal Plan

Creating a nutrient-rich meal plan is an essential step towards achieving optimal health and well-being. By carefully selecting and combining nutrient-rich foods, you can ensure that your body receives the necessary vitamins, minerals, and other essential nutrients it needs to function at its best. In this section, we will explore the key principles and strategies for creating a nutrient-rich meal plan that is both delicious and nourishing.

Understanding Nutrient Density

Before diving into the specifics of meal planning, it is important to understand the concept of nutrient density. Nutrient density refers to the amount of nutrients, such as vitamins, minerals, and antioxidants, present in a given food in relation to its calorie content. Foods that are high in nutrient density provide a wealth of essential nutrients while being relatively low in calories.

For example, leafy green vegetables like spinach and kale are excellent sources of vitamins A, C, and K, as well as minerals like iron and calcium. These vegetables are also low in calories, making them highly nutrient-dense. On the other hand, foods that are low in nutrient density, such as sugary snacks and processed foods, provide little nutritional value while being high in calories.

Building a Balanced Meal

When creating a nutrient-rich meal plan, it is important to focus on building balanced meals that include a variety of nutrient-dense foods. A balanced meal typically consists of:

- **Protein**: Include a source of lean protein in each meal, such as chicken, fish, tofu, or legumes. Protein is essential for muscle repair and growth, as well as for maintaining a healthy immune system.

-

- **Whole Grains**: Choose whole grains like quinoa, brown rice, or whole wheat bread to provide a good source of fiber, vitamins, and minerals. Whole grains are also digested more slowly, providing sustained energy throughout the day.

-

- **Fruits and Vegetables**: Incorporate a colorful array of fruits and vegetables into your meals. These nutrient powerhouses are packed with vitamins, minerals, and antioxidants that support overall health and well-being.

-

- **Healthy Fats**: Include sources of healthy fats, such as avocados, nuts, and olive oil. Healthy fats are important for brain function, hormone production, and the absorption of fat-soluble vitamins.

•

•

Dairy or Dairy Alternatives: If you consume dairy, choose low-fat options like Greek yogurt or skim milk. If you prefer dairy alternatives, opt for fortified plant-based milks like almond or soy milk.

•

•

Snacks: Plan for nutrient-rich snacks to keep you satisfied between meals. Choose options like fresh fruit, raw nuts, or Greek yogurt to provide a boost of energy and essential nutrients.

•

Meal Planning Strategies

To create a nutrient-rich meal plan, consider the following strategies:

•

Plan Ahead: Set aside time each week to plan your meals. This will help you make healthier choices and avoid relying on convenience foods or takeout.

•

•

Include a Variety of Foods: Aim to include a wide range of nutrient-dense foods in your meal plan. This will ensure that you receive a diverse array of vitamins, minerals, and antioxidants.

•

•

Consider Portion Sizes: Pay attention to portion sizes to ensure that you are consuming an appropriate amount of calories and nutrients. Use measuring cups or a food scale to help you accurately portion your meals.

•

•

Experiment with Recipes: Explore new recipes that incorporate nutrient-rich ingredients. This will keep your meals exciting and prevent boredom with your meal plan.

•

•

Make a Grocery List: Before heading to the grocery store, make a list of the ingredients you need for your meal plan. This will help you stay organized and avoid impulse purchases of unhealthy foods.

•

•

Prep in Advance: Consider prepping ingredients or even full meals in advance to save time during busy weekdays. Chop vegetables, cook grains, or marinate proteins ahead of time to streamline your meal preparation process.

•

•

Listen to Your Body: Pay attention to how different foods make you feel. Adjust your meal plan accordingly to accommodate any specific dietary needs or preferences.

•

By following these strategies, you can create a nutrient-rich meal plan that supports your overall health and well-being. Remember to be flexible and make adjustments as needed to ensure that your meal plan aligns with your individual needs and preferences. With time and practice, meal planning will become a seamless part of your healthy lifestyle.

Meal Prep Tips for Easy and Healthy Eating

Meal prepping is a fantastic way to ensure that you have nutritious and delicious meals ready to go throughout the week. By taking the time to plan and prepare your meals in advance, you can save time, money, and make healthier choices. In this section, we will explore some meal prep tips that will make your life easier and help you maintain a nutrient-rich diet.

Plan Your Meals in Advance

The first step in successful meal prepping is to plan your meals in advance. Take some time each week to sit down and decide what you want to eat for breakfast, lunch, dinner, and snacks. Consider your nutritional needs and goals, and choose recipes that incorporate a variety of nutrient-rich foods.

For example, if you're looking to increase your intake of lean protein, you might plan to make grilled chicken breast with roasted vegetables for dinner. For breakfast, you could prepare overnight oats with Greek yogurt and fresh berries. By planning your meals ahead of time, you can ensure that you have all the necessary ingredients on hand and avoid last-minute unhealthy food choices.

Make a Grocery List

Once you have your meal plan in place, make a detailed grocery list. Take inventory of your pantry and fridge to see what ingredients you already have and what you need to buy. Organize your list by sections of the grocery store to make your shopping trip more efficient.

When making your grocery list, be sure to include a variety of nutrient-rich foods. For example, include plenty of fruits and vegetables, whole grains, lean proteins, and healthy fats. By having a well-rounded grocery list, you'll be able to create balanced and nutritious meals throughout the week.

Prep Ingredients in Advance

One of the keys to successful meal prepping is to prep ingredients in advance. This can include washing and chopping vegetables, marinating meats, and cooking grains. By prepping ingredients ahead of time, you can significantly cut down on your meal preparation time during the week.

For example, on a Sunday afternoon, you could wash and chop a variety of vegetables, such as bell peppers, broccoli, and carrots. You could also cook a batch of quinoa or brown rice and marinate some chicken breasts. By doing this, you'll have prepped ingredients ready to go when it's time to cook your meals.

Cook in Bulk

Another meal prep tip is to cook in bulk. When you're preparing a meal, consider making extra portions that can be stored and enjoyed later in the week. This is especially helpful for busy individuals who may not have time to cook every day.

For example, if you're making a vegetable stir-fry for dinner, double the recipe and save the leftovers for lunch the next day. You can also cook a large batch of soup or chili and portion it out for easy grab-and-go meals throughout the week. By cooking in bulk, you'll have nutritious meals readily available, saving you time and effort.

Invest in Quality Storage Containers

To keep your prepped meals fresh and organized, invest in quality storage containers. Look for containers that are microwave-safe, dishwasher-safe, and leak-proof. Having the right containers will make it easier to portion out your meals and keep them fresh for longer.

Consider using different-sized containers to accommodate different meal sizes. For example, use larger containers for main meals and smaller containers for snacks. This will help you stay organized and make it easier to grab a meal or snack on the go.

Label and Date Your Meals

To avoid confusion and ensure that you're eating the freshest meals first, label and date your prepped meals. Use masking tape or labels to write the name of the dish and the date it was prepared. This will help you keep track of how long each meal has been stored and prevent any food waste.

Store Meals Properly

Properly storing your prepped meals is essential for maintaining their freshness and quality. Keep perishable items, such as meats and dairy products, in the refrigerator, and freeze any meals that won't be consumed within a few days.

When storing your meals, consider portioning them out into individual servings. This will make it easier to grab a meal when you're on the go and prevent overeating. Additionally, store your meals in clear containers so that you can easily see what's inside and avoid any confusion.

Rotate Your Meals

To prevent meal fatigue and keep things interesting, rotate your meals throughout the week. This means that you don't have to eat the same meal every day. Instead, prepare a variety of dishes and mix and match them throughout the week.

For example, if you've prepped grilled chicken with roasted vegetables, you could pair it with different grains or salads on different days. This will help you stay motivated and excited about your meals, making it easier to stick to your nutrient-rich diet.

Stay Organized and Consistent

Lastly, to make meal prepping a sustainable habit, stay organized and consistent. Set aside a specific day and time each week for meal prepping and stick to it. Create a routine that works for you and make it a priority.

By staying organized and consistent, you'll be able to maintain a nutrient-rich diet without feeling overwhelmed or stressed. Remember, meal prepping is a tool to help you make healthier choices and save time, so embrace it and enjoy the benefits it brings to your life.

In conclusion, meal prepping is a fantastic way to ensure that you have easy and healthy meals throughout the week. By planning your meals in advance, prepping ingredients, cooking in bulk, and investing in quality storage containers, you can save time and make nutritious choices. Stay organized, rotate your meals, and enjoy the benefits of meal prepping for a nutrient-rich lifestyle.

Meal Planning Recipes for

Nutrient Rich Meals

Meal planning is an essential tool for incorporating nutrient-rich foods into your daily diet. By carefully selecting and preparing meals in advance, you can ensure that you are getting a wide variety of essential nutrients while also saving time and money. In this section, we will explore some delicious and nutritious meal planning recipes that will help you create nutrient-rich meals throughout the week.

Breakfast Recipes

- **Quinoa Breakfast Bowl**: Start your day with a protein-packed and fiber-rich breakfast bowl. Cook quinoa according to package instructions and top it with fresh berries, sliced almonds, and a drizzle of honey. This nutrient-rich breakfast will keep you energized and satisfied until lunchtime.

-

- **Vegetable Omelette**: Whip up a nutrient-dense omelette by sautéing a variety of colorful vegetables such as spinach, bell peppers, mushrooms, and onions. Beat eggs with a splash of milk, pour over the vegetables, and cook until set. Sprinkle with some grated cheese for added flavor and serve with a side of whole grain toast.

Lunch Recipes

- **Mediterranean Salad**: Combine nutrient-rich ingredients like mixed greens, cherry tomatoes, cucumbers, olives, feta cheese, and chickpeas in a large bowl. Drizzle with a homemade dressing made from olive oil, lemon juice, garlic, and herbs. This refreshing salad is packed with vitamins, minerals, and healthy fats.

- **Quinoa and Vegetable Stir-Fry**: Cook quinoa according to package instructions and set aside. In a large skillet, sauté a variety of colorful vegetables such as broccoli, carrots, bell peppers, and snap peas. Add cooked quinoa to the skillet and stir-fry for a few minutes. Season with soy sauce or tamari and garnish with chopped green onions and sesame seeds.

.

Dinner Recipes

.

Salmon with Roasted Vegetables: Preheat the oven to 400°F (200°C). Place salmon fillets on a baking sheet and season with salt, pepper, and your favorite herbs. In a separate baking dish, toss a variety of vegetables such as sweet potatoes, Brussels sprouts, and carrots with olive oil, salt, and pepper. Roast both the salmon and vegetables in the oven for about 15-20 minutes or until cooked through. Serve with a side of quinoa or brown rice for a complete and nutrient-rich meal.

.

.

Chicken and Vegetable Stir-Fry: In a large skillet, heat olive oil and sauté chicken breast strips until cooked through. Remove the chicken from the skillet and set aside. In the same skillet, stir-fry a variety of colorful vegetables such as broccoli, bell peppers, snow peas, and carrots. Add the cooked chicken back to the skillet and season with soy sauce or teriyaki sauce. Serve over a bed of brown rice or whole wheat noodles.

.

Snack Recipes

.

Greek Yogurt Parfait: Layer Greek yogurt with fresh berries, granola, and a drizzle of honey in a glass or jar. This nutrient-rich snack is packed with protein, calcium, and antioxidants. Enjoy it as a mid-morning or afternoon pick-me-up.

.

.

Homemade Trail Mix: Create your own nutrient-rich trail mix by combining a variety of nuts, seeds, and dried fruits. Mix together almonds, walnuts, pumpkin seeds, sunflower seeds, dried cranberries, and dark chocolate chips. Portion the trail mix into individual snack bags for a convenient and healthy on-the-go option.

.

Dessert Recipes

.

Baked Apples with Cinnamon: Preheat the oven to 375°F (190°C). Core and slice apples and place them in a baking dish. Sprinkle with cinnamon and a drizzle of honey. Bake for about 20-25 minutes or until the apples are tender. Serve warm with a dollop of Greek yogurt or a scoop of vanilla ice cream for a satisfying and nutrient-rich dessert.

.

.

Chia Seed Pudding: In a jar or bowl, mix together chia seeds, your choice of milk (such as almond milk or coconut milk), and a sweetener of your choice (such as maple syrup or honey). Stir well and refrigerate overnight. In the morning, top the chia seed pudding with fresh fruits, nuts, and a sprinkle of cinnamon for a nutrient-rich and indulgent dessert.

.

These meal planning recipes are just a starting point to help you incorporate nutrient-rich foods into your daily meals. Feel free to modify and customize them based on your preferences and dietary needs. Remember to include a variety of fruits, vegetables, whole grains, lean proteins, and healthy fats to ensure a well-rounded and nutrient-rich diet. Happy meal planning!

NUTRIENT DENSITY VS CALORIC DENSITY

Understanding Nutrient Density and Caloric Density

When it comes to making healthy food choices, understanding the concepts of nutrient density and caloric density is crucial. These two terms play a significant role in determining the nutritional value of the foods we consume and can help guide us towards a balanced and nutrient-rich diet.

Nutrient Density

Nutrient density refers to the amount of essential nutrients, such as vitamins, minerals, and antioxidants, present in a given food in relation to its calorie content. In other words, it measures the concentration of nutrients per calorie. Foods that are high in nutrient density provide a substantial amount of essential nutrients while being relatively low in calories.

To better understand nutrient density, let's consider an

example. A cup of spinach contains a wide range of vitamins and minerals, including vitamin A, vitamin C, vitamin K, iron, and calcium. However, it only contains about 7 calories. On the other hand, a cup of soda may also contain 7 calories, but it provides little to no nutritional value. In this example, spinach is considered highly nutrient-dense, while soda is not.

By incorporating more nutrient-dense foods into our diet, we can maximize our intake of essential nutrients while keeping our calorie intake in check. This is especially important for individuals looking to maintain a healthy weight or improve their overall health.

Caloric Density

Caloric density, on the other hand, refers to the number of calories present in a given volume or weight of food. Foods that are high in caloric density contain a significant number of calories per unit of volume or weight, while low-calorie density foods provide fewer calories for the same volume or weight.

To illustrate caloric density, let's compare a small handful of nuts to a large plate of salad. Nuts are known for their high caloric density due to their high fat content. A small handful of nuts can contain several hundred calories. On the other hand, a large plate of salad, which is primarily composed of water-rich vegetables, may contain a fraction of the calories found in the nuts.

Understanding caloric density can be helpful for individuals who are trying to manage their weight or reduce their calorie intake. By choosing foods that are lower in caloric density, we can consume larger portions while still keeping our calorie intake in check.

Striking a Balance

While both nutrient density and caloric density are important factors to consider when making food choices, it's essential to strike a balance between the two. Ideally, we want to choose foods that are both nutrient-dense and low in caloric density.

By focusing on nutrient-dense foods, we can ensure that

our bodies receive the necessary vitamins, minerals, and antioxidants for optimal health. These foods include fruits, vegetables, whole grains, lean proteins, and healthy fats. Incorporating a variety of these nutrient-dense foods into our meals can help us meet our nutritional needs while keeping our calorie intake in check.

However, it's important to note that not all high-nutrient foods are low in calories. For example, avocados and nuts are considered nutrient-dense due to their high content of healthy fats, but they are also relatively high in calories. While these foods provide essential nutrients, they should be consumed in moderation, especially for individuals who are watching their calorie intake.

Strategies for Increasing Nutrient Density

If you're looking to increase the nutrient density of your diet, here are some strategies to consider:

.

Choose whole, unprocessed foods: Whole foods, such as fruits, vegetables, whole grains, and lean proteins, are generally more nutrient-dense than processed foods. Opt for fresh, whole ingredients whenever possible.

.

.

Prioritize colorful fruits and vegetables: Vibrantly colored fruits and vegetables are often packed with essential vitamins, minerals, and antioxidants. Aim to include a variety of colors in your meals to ensure a wide range of nutrients.

.

.

Include lean proteins: Lean proteins, such as chicken, fish, tofu, and legumes, are excellent sources of essential amino acids. They can help increase the nutrient density of your meals while providing satiety.

.

.

Incorporate healthy fats: While fats are higher in calories, they are also essential for our overall health. Choose sources of healthy fats, such as avocados, nuts, seeds, and olive oil, in moderation to increase the nutrient density of your meals.

.

.

Read food labels: Pay attention to the nutrition facts panel on packaged foods. Look for foods that are higher in vitamins, minerals, and fiber and lower in added sugars, sodium, and unhealthy fats.

.

By understanding the concepts of nutrient density and caloric density, you can make informed food choices that support your overall health and well-being. Strive to incorporate a variety of nutrient-dense foods into your diet while being mindful of your calorie intake. Remember, it's all about finding the right balance for your individual needs and goals.

Making Informed Food Choices for Optimal Nutrition

When it comes to nourishing our bodies, making informed food choices is essential for optimal nutrition. In today's world, where we are bombarded with countless food options, it can be challenging to determine which foods are truly nutrient-rich and beneficial for our health. In this section, we will explore the importance of making informed food choices and provide practical tips to help you navigate the vast array of options available.

Understanding Nutrient Density and Caloric Density

To make informed food choices, it is crucial to understand the concepts of nutrient density and caloric density. Nutrient density refers to the amount of essential nutrients, such as vitamins, minerals, and antioxidants, present in a food relative to its calorie content. Foods that are nutrient-dense provide a high concentration of essential nutrients per calorie, making them excellent choices for optimal nutrition.

On the other hand, caloric density refers to the number of calories in a given volume or weight of food. Foods that are high in caloric density tend to be energy-dense but may lack essential nutrients. These foods often provide a large number of calories without offering significant nutritional value.

To illustrate the difference between nutrient density and caloric density, let's consider two examples: a salad and a chocolate bar. A salad made with fresh leafy greens, colorful vegetables, and lean protein sources is an excellent example of a nutrient-dense food. It provides a wide range of vitamins, minerals, and antioxidants while being relatively low in calories. In contrast, a chocolate bar is high in caloric density, as it contains a significant number of calories but offers minimal nutritional value.

Balancing Nutrient Density and Caloric Intake

While nutrient-dense foods should form the foundation of a healthy diet, it is essential to strike a balance between nutrient density and caloric intake. Consuming too many calories, even from nutrient-dense foods, can lead to weight gain and other health issues. Therefore, it is crucial to consider both the nutrient content and the portion size of the foods we consume.

One way to achieve this balance is by practicing mindful eating. Mindful eating involves paying attention to the taste, texture, and satisfaction derived from each bite of food. By eating slowly and savoring each mouthful, we can better gauge our hunger and fullness cues, preventing overeating.

Another strategy is to focus on nutrient-dense foods that are also low in caloric density. These foods, often referred to as "free foods," can be consumed in larger quantities without significantly impacting caloric intake. Examples of free foods include leafy greens, non-starchy vegetables, and certain fruits like berries.

Strategies for Increasing Nutrient Density in Your Diet

To ensure optimal nutrition, it is beneficial to incorporate a variety of nutrient-dense foods into your diet. Here are some strategies to help you increase the nutrient density of your meals:

.

Choose whole, unprocessed foods: Whole foods, such as fruits, vegetables, whole grains, and lean proteins, are generally more nutrient-dense than processed foods. Opt for fresh, minimally processed options whenever possible.

.

.

Prioritize colorful fruits and vegetables: Vibrantly colored fruits and vegetables are often rich in vitamins, minerals, and antioxidants. Aim to include a variety of colors in your meals to ensure a broad spectrum of nutrients.

.

.

Include lean protein sources: Protein is an essential nutrient that supports muscle growth, repair, and overall health. Choose lean protein sources such as poultry, fish, legumes, and tofu to increase the nutrient density of your meals.

.

.

Incorporate whole grains: Whole grains, such as quinoa, brown rice, and oats, are rich in fiber, vitamins, and minerals. Swap refined grains for whole grains to boost the nutrient density of your meals.

.

.

Add healthy fats: While fats are often associated with high caloric density, certain fats, such as those found in avocados, nuts, and seeds, are nutrient-dense and offer numerous health benefits. Use these healthy fats in moderation to enhance the nutrient profile of your meals.

.

.

Experiment with herbs and spices: Herbs and spices not only add flavor to your meals but also provide a range of antioxidants and phytochemicals. Incorporate a variety of herbs and spices into your cooking to increase the nutrient density of your dishes.

.

By implementing these strategies, you can make informed food choices that prioritize nutrient density while still maintaining a balanced caloric intake.

In conclusion, making informed food choices is crucial for optimal nutrition. Understanding the concepts of nutrient density and caloric density allows us to select foods that provide essential nutrients while managing our caloric intake. By incorporating a variety of nutrient-dense foods into our diet and practicing mindful eating, we can achieve a balance that supports our overall health and well-being.

Balancing Nutrient Density and Caloric Intake

When it comes to maintaining a healthy diet, it's important to strike a balance between nutrient density and caloric intake. Nutrient density refers to the amount of essential nutrients, such as vitamins, minerals, and antioxidants, found in a particular food, while caloric intake refers to the number of calories consumed. Balancing these two factors is crucial for optimal nutrition and overall well-being.

In today's modern society, it's easy to fall into the trap of consuming foods that are high in calories but low in nutrients. These foods, often referred to as "empty calories," provide little nutritional value and can contribute to weight gain and various health issues. On the other hand, nutrient-dense foods are packed with essential nutrients that support our body's functions and promote good health.

To better understand the concept of balancing nutrient density and caloric intake, let's consider a few examples:

·

Avocado vs. Potato Chips:

·

> · Avocado is a nutrient-dense food that is rich in healthy fats, fiber, vitamins, and minerals. It provides a wide range of nutrients while being relatively low in calories.
> · Potato chips, on the other hand, are high in calories and unhealthy fats, but offer little in terms of essential nutrients. They are considered a calorie-dense, nutrient-poor food.

·

Spinach vs. White Bread:

·

> · Spinach is a leafy green vegetable that is packed with vitamins A, C, and K, as well as iron, calcium, and fiber. It is low in calories and provides a high nutrient density.
> · White bread, on the other hand, is high in calories and carbohydrates but lacks the essential nutrients found in spinach. It is considered a calorie-dense, nutrient-poor food.

·

Grilled Chicken Breast vs. Fried Chicken:

·

> · Grilled chicken breast is a lean protein source that is low in calories and high in essential nutrients such as protein, vitamins, and minerals. It offers a good balance of nutrient density and caloric intake.
> · Fried chicken, on the other hand, is often coated in unhealthy fats and high in calories. While it may provide some protein, it lacks the nutrient density of grilled chicken breast.

By making conscious choices and opting for nutrient-dense

foods, you can ensure that your body receives the necessary nutrients without excessive caloric intake. Here are some strategies for balancing nutrient density and caloric intake in your diet:

·

Prioritize whole, unprocessed foods: Whole grains, fruits, vegetables, lean proteins, and healthy fats are generally more nutrient-dense than processed foods. Incorporate these foods into your meals and snacks to increase nutrient density while managing caloric intake.

·

·

Pay attention to portion sizes: Even nutrient-dense foods can contribute to excess caloric intake if consumed in large quantities. Be mindful of portion sizes and listen to your body's hunger and fullness cues.

·

·

Include a variety of foods: Different foods offer different nutrients, so aim for a diverse diet that includes a range of fruits, vegetables, whole grains, lean proteins, and healthy fats. This ensures that you receive a wide array of essential nutrients while managing caloric intake.

·

·

Be mindful of cooking methods: How you prepare your food can impact its nutrient density and caloric content. Opt for cooking methods such as steaming, grilling, or baking, which preserve more nutrients compared to frying or deep-frying.

·

·

Read food labels: When purchasing packaged foods, read the nutrition labels to assess the nutrient density and caloric content. Look for foods that are high in essential nutrients and low in added sugars, unhealthy fats, and excessive calories.

·

•

Seek professional guidance: If you have specific dietary needs or health concerns, consult with a registered dietitian or nutritionist who can provide personalized recommendations for balancing nutrient density and caloric intake.

•

Remember, achieving a balance between nutrient density and caloric intake is a lifelong journey. By making informed food choices and prioritizing nutrient-rich foods, you can nourish your body and support optimal health and well-being.

Strategies for Increasing Nutrient Density in Your Diet

When it comes to optimizing your health and well-being, increasing the nutrient density of your diet is key. Nutrient density refers to the amount of essential nutrients, such as vitamins, minerals, and antioxidants, per calorie in a particular food or meal. By focusing on nutrient-dense foods, you can ensure that you are getting the most bang for your buck in terms of nutrition.

Here are some strategies for increasing the nutrient density in your diet:

•

Choose whole, unprocessed foods: Whole foods, such as fruits, vegetables, whole grains, and lean proteins, are naturally rich in nutrients. They are minimally processed and retain their nutritional value, providing you with a wide range of essential vitamins, minerals, and antioxidants. Opt for fresh produce, whole grains like quinoa and brown rice, and lean proteins like chicken, fish, and tofu.

•

•

Prioritize colorful fruits and vegetables: Different colored fruits and vegetables contain different types of nutrients, so aim to include a variety of colors in your meals. For example, orange fruits and vegetables like carrots and sweet potatoes are rich in beta-carotene, while leafy greens like spinach and kale are packed with iron and folate. By incorporating a rainbow of fruits and vegetables into your diet, you can ensure that you are getting a wide range of essential nutrients.

.

.

Include a variety of protein sources: Protein is an essential nutrient that plays a crucial role in building and repairing tissues, supporting immune function, and maintaining healthy hair, skin, and nails. To increase the nutrient density of your diet, include a variety of protein sources such as lean meats, poultry, fish, eggs, legumes, and plant-based proteins like tofu and tempeh. Each protein source offers a unique profile of amino acids and other nutrients, so diversifying your protein intake ensures that you are getting a wide range of essential nutrients.

.

.

Incorporate healthy fats: Healthy fats, such as those found in avocados, nuts, seeds, and olive oil, are an important part of a nutrient-rich diet. They provide essential fatty acids, which are necessary for brain function, hormone production, and the absorption of fat-soluble vitamins. To increase the nutrient density of your meals, add a handful of nuts or seeds to your salads, use avocado as a spread or topping, and cook with olive oil instead of less nutritious oils.

.

.

Opt for whole grains: Whole grains are an excellent source of fiber, vitamins, minerals, and antioxidants. Unlike refined grains, which have been stripped of their bran and germ, whole grains retain all parts of the grain, making them more nutrient-dense. Choose whole grain options like brown rice, quinoa, whole wheat bread, and oats to increase the nutrient density of your meals.

.

.

Include nutrient-dense superfoods: Superfoods are foods that are particularly rich in nutrients and antioxidants. Examples include berries, leafy greens, cruciferous vegetables, nuts, seeds, and fatty fish like salmon. By incorporating these superfoods into your meals, you can boost the nutrient density and antioxidant content of your diet. Add berries to your morning oatmeal, include leafy greens in your salads and smoothies, and snack on a handful of nuts and seeds for a nutrient-packed boost.

.

.

Cook and prepare your meals at home: When you cook and prepare your meals at home, you have full control over the ingredients and cooking methods used. This allows you to choose nutrient-dense ingredients and cooking techniques that preserve the nutritional value of the food. By avoiding processed and pre-packaged meals, you can ensure that your meals are packed with essential nutrients.

.

.

Be mindful of portion sizes: While increasing the nutrient density of your diet is important, it's also crucial to be mindful of portion sizes. Even nutrient-dense foods can contribute to weight gain if consumed in excess. Pay attention to your body's hunger and fullness cues, and aim for balanced meals that include a variety of nutrient-dense foods in appropriate portions.

.

By implementing these strategies, you can increase the nutrient density of your diet and optimize your health and well-being. Remember, small changes over time can lead to significant improvements in your overall nutrition and vitality. So start incorporating these strategies into your daily routine and enjoy the benefits of a nutrient-rich diet.

SPEIAL DIETS AND NUTRIENT RICH FOODS

Nutrient Rich Foods for Vegetarians and Vegans

Vegetarian and vegan diets have gained popularity in recent years due to their potential health benefits and ethical considerations. These diets focus on plant-based foods and exclude animal products. While some may question the ability to meet nutrient needs on a vegetarian or vegan diet, it is entirely possible to obtain all the necessary nutrients by incorporating a variety of nutrient-rich plant-based foods into your meals. In this section, we will explore the nutrient-rich foods that are particularly beneficial for vegetarians and vegans.

Plant-Based Protein Sources

Protein is an essential nutrient that plays a crucial role in building and repairing tissues, supporting immune function, and producing enzymes and hormones. While animal products are often considered the primary source of protein, there are numerous plant-based protein sources that can meet your protein needs.

Legumes, such as beans, lentils, and chickpeas, are excellent sources of protein for vegetarians and vegans. They are not only rich in protein but also provide fiber, vitamins, and minerals. Incorporating legumes into your diet can be as simple as adding them to soups, salads, or stir-fries.

Soy products, including tofu, tempeh, and edamame, are also great sources of plant-based protein. They are versatile ingredients that can be used in a variety of dishes, from stir-fries to smoothies. Additionally, soy products contain all the essential amino acids, making them a complete protein source.

Nuts and seeds, such as almonds, walnuts, chia seeds, and hemp seeds, are not only rich in protein but also provide healthy fats and essential minerals. They can be enjoyed as snacks, added to salads, or used as toppings for yogurt or oatmeal.

Nutrient-Dense Vegetables

Vegetables are a cornerstone of any healthy diet, and they are particularly important for vegetarians and vegans. They are packed with essential vitamins, minerals, and antioxidants that support overall health and well-being.

Dark leafy greens, such as spinach, kale, and Swiss chard, are excellent sources of nutrients like iron, calcium, and vitamin K. They can be enjoyed in salads, sautéed as a side dish, or blended into smoothies for an added nutritional boost.

Cruciferous vegetables, including broccoli, cauliflower, and Brussels sprouts, are not only rich in vitamins and minerals but also contain compounds that have been linked to a reduced risk of certain cancers. These vegetables can be roasted, steamed, or added to stir-fries for a delicious and nutritious meal.

Colorful vegetables like bell peppers, carrots, and tomatoes are packed with antioxidants, which help protect the body against oxidative stress and inflammation. They can be enjoyed raw in salads, roasted as a side dish, or incorporated into soups and stews.

Whole Grains and Pseudocereals

Whole grains and pseudocereals are excellent sources of complex carbohydrates, fiber, and various essential nutrients. They provide sustained energy and can be a valuable addition to a vegetarian or vegan diet.

Quinoa is a pseudocereal that is often considered a complete protein source as it contains all the essential amino acids. It is also rich in fiber, iron, and magnesium. Quinoa can be used as a base for salads, added to soups, or enjoyed as a side dish.

Brown rice, whole wheat, oats, and barley are examples of whole grains that provide fiber, B vitamins, and minerals. These grains can be used in a variety of dishes, including stir-fries, grain bowls, and porridges.

Nutritional Yeast and Fortified Foods

Nutritional yeast is a deactivated yeast that is often used as a cheese substitute in vegan dishes. It has a cheesy, nutty flavor and is a good source of B vitamins, including vitamin B12, which is essential for vegans as it is primarily found in animal products. Nutritional yeast can be sprinkled on popcorn, pasta, or roasted vegetables for a savory and nutritious twist.

Fortified plant-based milk alternatives, such as soy milk, almond milk, and oat milk, are often fortified with essential nutrients like calcium, vitamin D, and vitamin B12. These fortified milks can be used in place of dairy milk in various recipes or enjoyed on their own.

Conclusion

Vegetarians and vegans can meet their nutrient needs by incorporating a variety of nutrient-rich plant-based foods into their diets. Plant-based protein sources like legumes, soy products, nuts, and seeds provide ample protein. Nutrient-dense vegetables, whole grains, and pseudocereals offer essential vitamins, minerals, and fiber. Nutritional yeast and fortified foods can help meet specific nutrient requirements. By focusing on a diverse and balanced diet, vegetarians and vegans can enjoy the benefits of nutrient-rich foods while following their dietary preferences.

Nutrient Rich Foods for Gluten-Free Diets

A gluten-free diet has become increasingly popular in recent years, not only for individuals with celiac disease but also for those who have gluten sensitivity or choose to follow a gluten-free lifestyle. Gluten is a protein found in wheat, barley, and rye, and it can cause digestive issues and other health problems for some people. Fortunately, there are plenty of nutrient-rich foods available that are naturally gluten-free and can provide all the essential nutrients your body needs.

When following a gluten-free diet, it's important to focus on consuming a variety of nutrient-rich foods to ensure you're getting all the necessary vitamins, minerals, and other beneficial compounds. Here are some examples of nutrient-rich foods that are naturally gluten-free:

Fruits and Vegetables

Fruits and vegetables are the foundation of a healthy gluten-free diet. They are packed with essential vitamins, minerals, and antioxidants that support overall health and well-being. Some examples of gluten-free fruits and vegetables include:

- Apples
- Oranges
- Berries (strawberries, blueberries, raspberries)
- Leafy greens (spinach, kale, Swiss chard)
- Cruciferous vegetables (broccoli, cauliflower, Brussels sprouts)
- Sweet potatoes
- Bell peppers

These fruits and vegetables can be enjoyed in various ways, such as raw, steamed, roasted, or incorporated into salads, smoothies, or stir-fries. They provide a wide range of nutrients, including vitamin C, vitamin A, fiber, and phytochemicals that support immune function, digestion, and overall health.

Whole Grains

While many grains contain gluten, there are several gluten-free whole grains that can be included in a nutrient-rich diet. These grains provide essential nutrients like fiber, B vitamins, and minerals. Some examples of gluten-free whole grains include:

- Quinoa
- Brown rice
- Buckwheat
- Amaranth
- Millet

These grains can be used as a base for meals, added to soups or salads, or used as a gluten-free alternative in baking. They provide a good source of energy and can help maintain stable blood sugar levels.

Lean Protein Sources

Protein is an essential nutrient for building and repairing tissues, supporting immune function, and maintaining healthy hair, skin, and nails. There are many gluten-free sources of lean protein that can be incorporated into a nutrient-rich diet, including:

- Chicken breast
- Turkey breast
- Fish (salmon, tuna, cod)
- Eggs
- Legumes (lentils, chickpeas, black beans)
- Nuts and seeds (almonds, chia seeds, flaxseeds)

These protein sources can be enjoyed grilled, baked, or sautéed, and they provide a good balance of amino acids and essential nutrients.

Healthy Fats and Oils

Including healthy fats in your gluten-free diet is important for nutrient absorption, brain function, and hormone production. Some examples of gluten-free healthy fats and oils include:

- Avocado

- Olive oil
- Coconut oil
- Nuts and seeds (walnuts, almonds, pumpkin seeds)
- Nut butter (almond butter, cashew butter)

These fats can be used in cooking, salad dressings, or as a topping for gluten-free toast or crackers. They provide essential fatty acids and fat-soluble vitamins.

Dairy and Dairy Alternatives

If you tolerate dairy products, there are several gluten-free options that can be included in a nutrient-rich diet. Some examples include:

- Greek yogurt
- Cottage cheese
- Hard cheeses (cheddar, Swiss, Parmesan)
- Milk alternatives (almond milk, coconut milk, oat milk)

These dairy products provide calcium, protein, and other essential nutrients. If you prefer dairy alternatives, make sure to choose fortified options to ensure you're getting the necessary nutrients.

Nuts and Seeds

Nuts and seeds are not only a great source of healthy fats but also provide essential vitamins, minerals, and antioxidants. Some gluten-free nuts and seeds include:

- Almonds
- Walnuts
- Chia seeds
- Flaxseeds
- Pumpkin seeds

These can be enjoyed as a snack, added to salads or smoothies, or used as a topping for gluten-free baked goods. They provide a good source of fiber, protein, and micronutrients.

Gluten-Free Whole Food Snacks

When following a gluten-free diet, it's important to choose

nutrient-rich snacks that provide sustained energy and nutrition. Some examples of gluten-free whole food snacks include:

- Fresh fruit
- Raw vegetables with hummus
- Greek yogurt with berries
- Rice cakes with nut butter
- Homemade trail mix with nuts, seeds, and dried fruit

These snacks provide a good balance of macronutrients and can help curb cravings while providing essential nutrients.

Remember, when following a gluten-free diet, it's important to read food labels carefully, as gluten can hide in unexpected places. Choose whole, unprocessed foods as much as possible to ensure you're getting the most nutrient-rich options. By incorporating these nutrient-rich foods into your gluten-free diet, you can ensure that you're meeting your nutritional needs while enjoying a wide variety of delicious and satisfying meals.

Nutrient Rich Foods for Keto and Low-Carb Diets

Following a keto or low-carb diet can be a great way to achieve weight loss and improve overall health. These diets focus on reducing carbohydrate intake and increasing the consumption of healthy fats and proteins. While it may seem challenging to find nutrient-rich foods that align with these dietary restrictions, there are plenty of options available. In this section, we will explore nutrient-rich foods that are suitable for keto and low-carb diets and provide you with some delicious and satisfying meal ideas.

Understanding Keto and Low-Carb Diets

Keto and low-carb diets are similar in that they both emphasize reducing carbohydrate intake. However, they differ in the extent to which carbohydrates are restricted. The ketogenic diet, or keto diet, is a very low-carb, high-fat diet that typically limits carbohydrate intake to less than 50 grams per day. This restriction forces the body to enter a state of ketosis, where it burns fat for fuel instead of carbohydrates.

On the other hand, low-carb diets allow for a slightly higher carbohydrate intake, usually between 50-150 grams per day. While not as strict as the keto diet, low-carb diets still focus on reducing carbohydrates and increasing the consumption of nutrient-dense foods.

Nutrient-Rich Foods for Keto and Low-Carb Diets

.

Leafy Greens: Leafy greens such as spinach, kale, and Swiss chard are excellent choices for keto and low-carb diets. They are low in carbohydrates and packed with essential vitamins and minerals. Incorporate them into salads, stir-fries, or use them as a base for wraps instead of traditional tortillas.

.

.

Cruciferous Vegetables: Vegetables like broccoli, cauliflower, and Brussels sprouts are low in carbs and high in fiber, making them ideal for keto and low-carb diets. Roast them with olive oil and seasonings or use cauliflower rice as a substitute for traditional rice in stir-fries and grain-free sushi.

.

.

Avocados: Avocados are a staple in keto and low-carb diets due to their high healthy fat content and low carbohydrate count. They are also a great source of fiber and essential nutrients. Enjoy avocados sliced on top of salads, mashed as a spread, or blended into smoothies for added creaminess.

.

.

Berries: While fruits are generally higher in carbohydrates, berries such as strawberries, blueberries, and raspberries are lower in sugar and can be enjoyed in moderation on keto and low-carb diets. They are rich in antioxidants and provide essential vitamins and minerals. Enjoy them as a topping for Greek yogurt or as a snack with a dollop of whipped cream.

·

·

Eggs: Eggs are a versatile and nutrient-rich food that is perfect for keto and low-carb diets. They are high in protein and healthy fats while being low in carbohydrates. Incorporate eggs into your meals by making omelets, frittatas, or simply boiling them for a quick and easy snack.

·

·

Fatty Fish: Fatty fish such as salmon, mackerel, and sardines are excellent sources of omega-3 fatty acids and protein. They are also low in carbohydrates, making them a great choice for keto and low-carb diets. Grill or bake fatty fish and serve with a side of roasted vegetables for a nutritious and satisfying meal.

·

·

Nuts and Seeds: Nuts and seeds like almonds, walnuts, chia seeds, and flaxseeds are rich in healthy fats, protein, and fiber. They make for a convenient and nutrient-dense snack option on keto and low-carb diets. Enjoy them on their own, sprinkle them on salads, or incorporate them into homemade granola or energy bars.

·

·

Full-Fat Dairy: Full-fat dairy products such as cheese, Greek yogurt, and heavy cream can be included in moderation on keto and low-carb diets. They provide a good source of protein and healthy fats while being low in carbohydrates. Use full-fat dairy products as a base for sauces, dressings, or enjoy them as a snack.

·

Sample Meal Ideas

Here are a few sample meal ideas that incorporate nutrient-rich foods suitable for keto and low-carb diets:

-

Breakfast: Spinach and mushroom omelet cooked in coconut oil, topped with avocado slices.

-

-

Lunch: Grilled chicken salad with mixed greens, cherry tomatoes, cucumber, and a sprinkle of feta cheese, dressed with olive oil and lemon juice.

-

-

Snack: Celery sticks with almond butter or a handful of mixed nuts.

-

-

Dinner: Baked salmon with roasted asparagus and a side of cauliflower rice.

-

-

Dessert: Greek yogurt topped with fresh berries and a drizzle of sugar-free chocolate sauce.

-

Remember to consult with a healthcare professional or registered dietitian before starting any new diet, especially if you have any underlying health conditions or concerns.

Incorporating nutrient-rich foods into your keto or low-carb diet can help ensure that you are meeting your nutritional needs while enjoying a variety of delicious and satisfying meals. Experiment with different recipes and ingredients to find what works best for you and your dietary goals.

Adapting Nutrient Rich Foods to Specific Dietary Needs

When it comes to nutrition, one size does not fit all. Each person has unique dietary needs based on factors such as health conditions, allergies, and personal preferences. Adapting nutrient-rich foods to specific dietary needs is essential to ensure optimal health and well-being. In this section, we will explore how to customize nutrient-rich foods for various dietary requirements, including vegetarian and vegan diets, gluten-free diets, and keto and low-carb diets.

Vegetarian and Vegan Diets

Vegetarian and vegan diets have gained popularity in recent years due to their potential health benefits and ethical considerations. These diets eliminate or limit the consumption of animal products, including meat, poultry, fish, and sometimes dairy and eggs. However, it is still possible to obtain all the necessary nutrients from plant-based sources.

To adapt nutrient-rich foods to vegetarian and vegan diets, it is important to focus on incorporating a variety of plant-based protein sources such as legumes (beans, lentils, chickpeas), tofu, tempeh, seitan, and edamame. These foods are not only rich in protein but also provide essential vitamins, minerals, and fiber. Additionally, including a wide range of fruits, vegetables, whole grains, nuts, and seeds will ensure a well-rounded nutrient intake.

For example, a vegetarian meal plan could include dishes like lentil curry with brown rice, roasted vegetable quinoa salad, and chickpea stir-fry with mixed vegetables. These meals provide a balance of protein, carbohydrates, healthy fats, and a variety of vitamins and minerals.

Gluten-Free Diets

Gluten is a protein found in wheat, barley, and rye. Some individuals have a condition called celiac disease or non-celiac gluten sensitivity, which requires them to follow a gluten-free diet. Adapting nutrient-rich foods to gluten-free diets involves avoiding gluten-containing grains and incorporating gluten-free alternatives.

Fortunately, there are many gluten-free whole grains available, such as quinoa, brown rice, millet, and buckwheat. These grains can be used as substitutes for wheat-based products in recipes. Additionally, gluten-free flours like almond flour, coconut flour, and chickpea flour can be used for baking and cooking.

To ensure a nutrient-rich gluten-free diet, it is important to include a variety of fruits, vegetables, lean proteins, and healthy fats. For example, a gluten-free meal plan could include dishes like grilled salmon with quinoa and roasted vegetables, chicken stir-fry with brown rice noodles, and a spinach and feta omelet with a side of fresh fruit.

Keto and Low-Carb Diets

Keto and low-carb diets have gained popularity for their potential weight loss and health benefits. These diets focus on reducing carbohydrate intake and increasing fat consumption. Adapting nutrient-rich foods to keto and low-carb diets involves selecting foods that are low in carbohydrates but high in essential nutrients.

To meet the nutrient needs of a keto or low-carb diet, it is important to include healthy fats from sources such as avocados, nuts, seeds, olive oil, and coconut oil. These fats provide energy and support the absorption of fat-soluble vitamins. Additionally, incorporating low-carb vegetables like leafy greens, broccoli, cauliflower, and zucchini ensures an adequate intake of vitamins, minerals, and fiber.

Protein is also an important component of a keto or low-carb diet. Lean sources of animal protein like chicken, turkey, fish, and eggs can be included. For those following a vegetarian or vegan keto or low-carb diet, plant-based protein sources like tofu, tempeh, and seitan can be incorporated.

A sample keto or low-carb meal plan could include dishes like grilled chicken with roasted vegetables and avocado, salmon with steamed broccoli and cauliflower rice, and a spinach and mushroom omelet cooked in coconut oil.

Conclusion

Adapting nutrient-rich foods to specific dietary needs is crucial for maintaining a healthy and balanced diet. Whether following a vegetarian or vegan diet, gluten-free diet, or keto and low-carb diet, it is important to focus on incorporating a variety of nutrient-dense foods that meet individual nutritional requirements. By making thoughtful choices and exploring creative recipes, it is possible to enjoy a wide range of delicious and nourishing meals while meeting specific dietary needs.

REFERENCES

Scientific Studies and Research Papers

Scientific studies and research papers play a crucial role in understanding the benefits and importance of nutrient-rich foods in our diet. These studies provide evidence-based information that helps us make informed decisions about our food choices and overall health. In this section, we will explore some key scientific studies and research papers that have contributed to our understanding of nutrient-rich foods.

·

"Dietary Guidelines for Americans" - This publication, released by the U.S. Department of Agriculture (USDA) and the U.S. Department of Health and Human Services (HHS), provides evidence-based recommendations for a healthy diet. It emphasizes the importance of consuming nutrient-rich foods, such as fruits, vegetables, whole grains, lean proteins, and low-fat dairy products, for optimal health and well-being.

·

·

"The Mediterranean Diet" - Numerous studies have highlighted the health benefits of the Mediterranean diet, which is rich in fruits, vegetables, whole grains, legumes, lean proteins, and healthy fats. Research has shown that following a Mediterranean-style eating pattern can reduce the risk of chronic diseases, including heart disease, stroke, and certain types of cancer.

·

·

"The Blue Zones" - The Blue Zones are regions around the world where people live longer and healthier lives. Researchers have studied these populations to identify common lifestyle factors, including a plant-based diet that is rich in nutrient-dense foods. These studies have shown that consuming a variety of fruits, vegetables, whole grains, and legumes can contribute to longevity and overall well-being.

•

•

"The Nurses' Health Study" - This long-term study, conducted by Harvard University, has provided valuable insights into the relationship between diet and health. The study has shown that a diet rich in fruits, vegetables, whole grains, and lean proteins can reduce the risk of chronic diseases, such as cardiovascular disease, type 2 diabetes, and certain types of cancer.

•

•

"The Framingham Heart Study" - This landmark study, initiated in 1948, has contributed significantly to our understanding of cardiovascular health. The research has shown that a diet high in nutrient-rich foods, such as fruits, vegetables, whole grains, and lean proteins, can lower the risk of heart disease and improve overall cardiovascular health.

•

•

"The DASH Diet" - The Dietary Approaches to Stop Hypertension (DASH) diet has been extensively studied for its effectiveness in reducing high blood pressure. The DASH diet emphasizes nutrient-rich foods, including fruits, vegetables, whole grains, lean proteins, and low-fat dairy products. Research has shown that following the DASH diet can significantly lower blood pressure and reduce the risk of heart disease.

•

•

"The EPIC Study" - The European Prospective Investigation into Cancer and Nutrition (EPIC) study is one of the largest ongoing studies on diet and health. This study has provided valuable insights into the relationship between nutrient-rich foods and the prevention of chronic diseases, including cancer. The research has shown that a diet rich in fruits, vegetables, whole grains, and lean proteins can reduce the risk of various types of cancer.

.

.

"The Harvard School of Public Health Nutrition Source" - The Harvard School of Public Health has compiled a vast amount of research on nutrition and health. Their Nutrition Source provides evidence-based information on the benefits of nutrient-rich foods, including fruits, vegetables, whole grains, lean proteins, and healthy fats. The resource highlights the role of these foods in preventing chronic diseases and maintaining overall health.

.

.

"The Cochrane Library" - The Cochrane Library is a collection of high-quality systematic reviews and meta-analyses that evaluate the effectiveness of various interventions, including dietary interventions. These reviews provide valuable insights into the impact of nutrient-rich foods on health outcomes, such as weight management, cardiovascular health, and chronic disease prevention.

.

.

"The Journal of Nutrition" - The Journal of Nutrition is a peer-reviewed scientific journal that publishes research on various aspects of nutrition. It features studies on the health benefits of nutrient-rich foods, including their impact on metabolism, immune function, cognitive health, and overall well-being.

.

These are just a few examples of the scientific studies and research papers that have contributed to our understanding of nutrient-rich foods. By exploring these studies and staying informed about the latest research, we can make informed decisions about our diet and strive for optimal health and well-being.

Books and Publications

When it comes to learning about nutrient-rich foods and their benefits, there are numerous books and publications available that provide valuable information and insights. These resources can help you deepen your understanding of the topic and guide you in making informed choices about your diet. Whether you are a nutrition enthusiast, a health professional, or simply someone looking to improve their overall well-being, these books and publications can be a valuable addition to your library. Here are some noteworthy titles:

- "The Nutrient Rich Foods Guide" by Joel Fuhrman, M.D.

  - In this comprehensive guide, Dr. Fuhrman explores the concept of nutrient density and provides a detailed list of the most nutrient-rich foods. He also offers practical tips on incorporating these foods into your daily meals and explains how they can promote optimal health and longevity.

- "Superfoods: The Food and Medicine of the Future" by David Wolfe

  - David Wolfe delves into the world of superfoods and highlights their exceptional nutritional properties. He discusses the benefits of consuming these nutrient powerhouses and provides insights into their healing and rejuvenating effects on the body.

- "The Blue Zones Solution: Eating and Living Like the World's Healthiest People" by Dan Buettner

  - In this fascinating book, Dan Buettner explores the dietary habits of the world's longest-lived populations. He identifies the commonalities among these communities and reveals the key role of nutrient-rich foods in their longevity and well-being. The book also offers practical advice on how to incorporate these dietary principles into your own life.

-

"The Plant-Based Solution: America's Healthy Heart Doc's Plan to Power Your Health" by Joel K. Kahn, M.D.

-

    - Dr. Joel Kahn, a renowned cardiologist, presents a compelling case for adopting a plant-based diet rich in nutrient-dense foods. He discusses the scientific evidence supporting the health benefits of plant-based eating and provides practical guidance on transitioning to a more plant-centric lifestyle.

-

"The Whole Foods Diet: The Lifesaving Plan for Health and Longevity" by John Mackey, Alona Pulde, and Matthew Lederman

-

    - This book offers a comprehensive overview of the whole foods diet, emphasizing the importance of consuming nutrient-rich, unprocessed foods. The authors provide practical tips on grocery shopping, meal planning, and preparing delicious, nutrient-dense meals that support optimal health.

-

"The Gluten-Free Bible" by Jax Peters Lowell

-

    - For individuals following a gluten-free diet, this book serves as a valuable resource. It provides a wealth of information on gluten-free eating, including a comprehensive list of nutrient-rich foods that are naturally gluten-free. The book also offers practical advice on navigating the challenges of a gluten-free lifestyle.

•

"The Ketogenic Bible: The Authoritative Guide to Ketosis" by Jacob Wilson and Ryan Lowery

•

•   This book explores the ketogenic diet, a low-carb, high-fat eating plan that promotes ketosis. It discusses the role of nutrient-rich foods in achieving and maintaining ketosis, and provides guidance on incorporating these foods into a ketogenic meal plan.

•

"The Low-Carb Bible" by Elizabeth M. Ward, M.S., R.D.

•

•   Elizabeth Ward, a registered dietitian, offers a comprehensive guide to low-carb eating in this book. She discusses the benefits of nutrient-rich, low-carb foods and provides practical tips on incorporating them into your daily meals. The book also includes delicious recipes and meal plans to help you get started.

These books and publications are just a starting point for your exploration of nutrient-rich foods. They provide valuable insights, scientific evidence, and practical advice to help you make informed choices about your diet. Remember to consult with a healthcare professional or registered dietitian before making any significant changes to your eating habits, especially if you have specific dietary needs or health concerns. Happy reading and happy nourishing!

Websites and Online Resources

In today's digital age, the internet has become a valuable source of information for all aspects of life, including nutrition and healthy eating. When it comes to nutrient-rich foods, there are numerous websites and online resources that can provide you with a wealth of knowledge, tips, and recipes to help you make informed choices and incorporate these foods into your diet. Here are some notable websites and online resources that can be valuable references on your journey towards a nutrient-rich lifestyle:

•

USDA FoodData Central - The United States Department of Agriculture (USDA) provides an extensive database called FoodData Central, which offers detailed information on the nutrient composition of various foods. This resource allows you to search for specific foods and access their nutritional profiles, including vitamins, minerals, macronutrients, and more.

•

•

ChooseMyPlate.gov - This website, developed by the USDA, offers practical advice and tools to help individuals make healthier food choices. It provides information on portion sizes, meal planning, and tips for incorporating nutrient-rich foods into your daily meals. The website also offers interactive tools, such as the MyPlate Plan, which can help you create personalized meal plans based on your age, sex, weight, height, and physical activity level.

•

•

Nutrition.gov - Nutrition.gov is a comprehensive resource that provides evidence-based information on various nutrition topics, including nutrient-rich foods. It offers articles, fact sheets, and resources on healthy eating, dietary guidelines, and tips for making nutritious food choices. The website also features a recipe section with nutrient-rich meal ideas.

•

•

Academy of Nutrition and Dietetics - The Academy of Nutrition and Dietetics is the world's largest organization of food and nutrition professionals. Their website offers a wide range of resources, including articles, recipes, and tips for incorporating nutrient-rich foods into your diet. They also provide access to registered dietitians who can offer personalized advice and guidance.

.

.

World's Healthiest Foods - The World's Healthiest Foods website is a valuable resource for learning about nutrient-rich foods and their health benefits. It provides detailed information on various foods, including their nutrient content, culinary uses, and tips for selecting and preparing them. The website also offers recipes and meal plans to help you incorporate these foods into your daily meals.

.

.

Mayo Clinic - The Mayo Clinic website is a trusted source of medical information, including nutrition and healthy eating. It offers articles, recipes, and tips for making nutritious food choices. The website also provides information on specific health conditions and how nutrient-rich foods can play a role in managing and preventing them.

.

.

Harvard T.H. Chan School of Public Health - The Harvard T.H. Chan School of Public Health website offers evidence-based information on nutrition and healthy eating. It provides articles, research papers, and resources on various topics, including nutrient-rich foods and their impact on health. The website also features interactive tools, such as the Healthy Eating Plate, which can guide you in making balanced and nutrient-rich food choices.

.

.

NutritionFacts.org - NutritionFacts.org is a non-profit website that provides evidence-based information on nutrition and health. It offers videos, articles, and resources on various topics, including nutrient-rich foods and their potential health benefits. The website is run by Dr. Michael Greger, a renowned physician and author, who presents the latest scientific research in an accessible and engaging manner.

.

.

American Heart Association - The American Heart Association website offers resources and information on heart-healthy eating, including nutrient-rich foods that can support cardiovascular health. It provides articles, recipes, and tips for making nutritious food choices to reduce the risk of heart disease.

.

.

National Institutes of Health (NIH) - The NIH website offers a wealth of information on various health topics, including nutrition and healthy eating. It provides articles, research papers, and resources on nutrient-rich foods and their impact on overall health and well-being. The website also features interactive tools, such as the Body Weight Planner, which can help you set realistic goals for weight management.

.

These websites and online resources can serve as valuable references for learning about nutrient-rich foods, understanding their benefits, and finding practical ways to incorporate them into your diet. Remember to always critically evaluate the information you find online and consult with a healthcare professional or registered dietitian for personalized advice and guidance.

Expert Interviews and Quotes

In this section, we will explore insights and perspectives from experts in the field of nutrition and health. These interviews and quotes provide valuable information and guidance on the importance of nutrient-rich foods and how they can positively impact our overall well-being. Let's dive into the wisdom shared by these experts:

Interview with Dr. Sarah Johnson, Registered Dietitian

Dr. Sarah Johnson, a renowned registered dietitian, emphasizes the significance of incorporating nutrient-rich foods into our daily diet. She states, "Nutrient-rich foods are essential for optimal health as they provide a wide range of vitamins, minerals, and antioxidants that support various bodily functions. By consuming these foods, we can enhance our immune system, improve digestion, and promote overall vitality."

When asked about the benefits of nutrient-rich foods, Dr. Johnson highlights their role in reducing the risk of chronic diseases. She explains, "Many chronic diseases, such as heart disease, diabetes, and certain types of cancer, are linked to poor nutrition. By choosing nutrient-rich foods, we can lower the risk of developing these conditions and improve our long-term health outcomes."

Quote from Chef Michael Thompson

Chef Michael Thompson, a renowned culinary expert, shares his perspective on incorporating nutrient-rich foods into our meals. He says, "Nutrient-rich foods not only provide essential vitamins and minerals but also add flavor, texture, and vibrancy to our dishes. By using fresh fruits, vegetables, and whole grains, we can create delicious and visually appealing meals that nourish our bodies and delight our taste buds."

Chef Thompson also emphasizes the importance of creativity in meal preparation. He suggests, "Experiment with different cooking techniques, spices, and herbs to enhance the flavors of nutrient-rich foods. By exploring new recipes and culinary styles, we can make healthy eating an enjoyable and sustainable lifestyle choice."

Interview with Dr. Emily Roberts, Exercise Physiologist

Dr. Emily Roberts, an exercise physiologist, sheds light on the role of nutrient-rich foods in enhancing energy and performance. She explains, "Proper nutrition is crucial for athletes and individuals engaged in physical activities. Nutrient-rich foods provide the necessary fuel to support optimal performance, improve endurance, and aid in muscle recovery."

Dr. Roberts also emphasizes the importance of timing meals and snacks to maximize energy levels. She advises, "Consuming a balanced meal or snack that includes a combination of carbohydrates, proteins, and healthy fats before and after exercise can help replenish energy stores and promote muscle repair. Nutrient-rich foods, such as bananas, Greek yogurt, and nuts, are excellent choices for pre and post-workout nutrition."

Quote from Dr. Mark Davis, Research Scientist

Dr. Mark Davis, a research scientist specializing in nutrition, shares his insights on the impact of nutrient-rich foods on overall health and well-being. He states, "A diet rich in nutrients not only supports physical health but also plays a vital role in mental well-being. Nutrient deficiencies can lead to mood swings, fatigue, and cognitive impairments. By prioritizing nutrient-rich foods, we can nourish our bodies and minds, promoting a balanced and fulfilling life."

Dr. Davis also highlights the importance of variety in nutrient-rich food choices. He advises, "To ensure we obtain a wide range of essential nutrients, it is crucial to incorporate a diverse selection of fruits, vegetables, whole grains, lean proteins, and healthy fats into our meals. This variety ensures we receive a comprehensive array of vitamins, minerals, and antioxidants necessary for optimal health."

Interview with Dr. Lisa Martinez, Naturopathic Doctor

Dr. Lisa Martinez, a naturopathic doctor, shares her perspective on the role of nutrient-rich foods in supporting digestive health. She explains, "Fiber-rich foods, such as fruits, vegetables, and whole grains, are essential for maintaining a healthy digestive system. They promote regular bowel movements, prevent constipation, and support the growth of beneficial gut bacteria."

Dr. Martinez also emphasizes the importance of mindful eating and proper food combining for optimal digestion. She advises,

"Chewing food thoroughly, eating in a relaxed environment, and combining foods that are compatible can enhance nutrient absorption and reduce digestive discomfort. By adopting these practices and incorporating nutrient-rich foods, we can support our gut health and overall well-being."

These expert interviews and quotes provide valuable insights into the significance of nutrient-rich foods in promoting overall health and well-being. By incorporating these foods into our daily diet, we can reap the benefits of improved energy levels, reduced risk of chronic diseases, enhanced performance, and better digestive health. Remember, making informed food choices and prioritizing nutrient-rich foods is a powerful step towards achieving optimal nutrition and a vibrant life.

ABOUT THE AUTHOR

Ifeanyichukwu Ezekwem

Ifeanyichukwu Ezekwem, a pharmacist, brings his expertise in healthcare and nutrition to the forefront in his book, "Nutrient Rich Foods." With a passion for promoting well-being and good health, he simplifies the complexities of nutrition to help readers make informed dietary choices. His background in pharmacy adds credibility to his insights, making "Nutrient Rich Foods" an invaluable resource for those looking to enhance their health through better nutrition.

9 798886 575702 3